The Pilates Reformer

A Manual For Instructors

By Marci Clark, BS
Christine Romani-Ruby MPT, ATC

The Pilates Reformer

A Manual For Instructors

By Marci Clark, BS
Christine Romani-Ruby MPT, ATC

© Copyright PowerHouse Pilates, LLC

Printed in the United States of America

ISBN: 1-891231-45-6
Library of Congress Control Number: 200108934

Word Association Publishers
205 Fifth Avenue
Tarentum, Pennsylvania 15084
800-827-7903
www.wordassociation.com

Table of Contents

The Pillars of Joseph H. Pilates' Principles

Beginner Reformer Exercises

Intermediate Reformer Exercises

Advanced Reformer Exercises

Beginning Your Own Pilates Program

Glossary

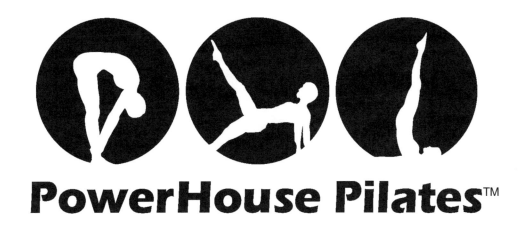

Reformer Encyclopedia

Special thanks to:

Our families for their patience in our absence as we created this manual: Mike Matteo, Craig Ruby, Cassandra Ruby, and Chloe Ruby,

And to David Littman of Balanced Body for his support and encouragement.

And to Ken Endelman of Balanced Body for freeing the word Pilates and for the fine equipment on which we perform our work.

And to Kathleen Waters-Harper for her technical advice and Pilates expertise.

And to The PowerHouse Institute Staff for their hard work and proofreading skills.

Introduction

Welcome to the PowerHouse Institute Reformer Manual for fitness professionals. Joseph Pilates states in his book, *Your Health,* written in 1920 "that this exercise will be what people want and need in the new millennium." Sure enough, the new millennium has arrived and Pilates is the newest fitness craze. Fitness professionals now find themselves challenged with learning these new techniques to meet the demands of their clients.

This manual was created to illustrate basic and intermediate reformer exercises in a fitness format for use in a group exercise class. Each exercise is broken down into categories from benefits to set up and movement. Safety prerequisites and cues are also included to enhance teacher skills. It is recommended that this manual is used in combination with formal Pilates training by The PowerHouse Institute.

For more information on
The PowerHouse Institute Pilates Training
visit our website **www.powerhouseinstitute.com**
or call toll free
1-877-716-4879

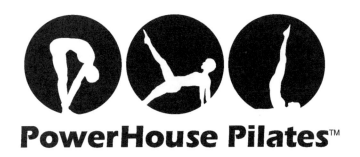

PowerHouse Pilates™

THE PILLARS OF JOSEPH H. PILATES' PRINCIPLES

Joseph Hubertus Pilates   1880-1967

"This will be the exercise that people will want and need in the new millennium," wrote Joseph Pilates in his book *Your Health in 1920*. We shuddered as we read this statement when we were first introduced to Contrology (what Joseph called his Pilates method). How did Joseph know that as the new millennium approached both fitness and rehabilitation would be focusing on core exercise or what Joseph called the Powerhouse?

Active in both fitness and rehabilitation for 15 years, the Pilates method has tied our two worlds together. Wanting desperately to teach the fitness crowds about posture and functional strength and get the rehabilitating patients into a fitness regimen, we finally found the answer. Pilates exercise could accommodate and challenge all levels from the injured to the elite athlete and could create profound results.

As fitness professionals, we were now able to meet the demands of the 90s not just to lose weight and look good but to feel good, stand taller, perform better, and prevent illness. As rehabilitation professionals, we had a whole new box of tools to get the results that the patients needed to progress into a fitness routine.

Joseph Pilates was before his time. Maybe it was because he was ill himself, or because he worked with so many injured bodies. He came to understand movement and stability in the body at a level that we are just scientifically mastering today. We often say that Joseph was doing Physical Therapy without knowing the "whys". He just knew his method worked and it still does.

Now that the word Pilates has become public domain and the benefits of the exercises have been demonstrated by famous personalities, we are seeing a growth of its popularity. With this growth, there will be many levels of Pilates instruction and many new environments created for Pilates exercise.

One of the newest environments is the group reformer class for which this book was written. The group reformer class creates an affordable fitness environment for Pilates exercise. In this environment we expect to see the client transform at a slower rate. However, the pace is just as effective as a private session. Incorporated within it are the many benefits of the group setting that we are so accustomed to in fitness, as well as the personal attention of a private Pilates session. In these classes, the instructor must make adjustments to accommodate many exercise levels. This class is truly a cross between personal training and group exercise. We have entitled our classes group personal training on the Pilates reformer.

As these new environments are created we must remember to maintain the many principles of Joseph's work. As fitness professionals, your background in anatomy and fitness are an asset, but remember that attention to form and detail, low repetition, emphasis on the process not the result are the underpinnings of Joseph's method. Stay within the limits of your practice and base your teaching skills not on hours or certification, but on experience and client success.

Benefits of the Pilates exercise program

1. Increases muscle strength, joint mobility, flexibility and muscle balance
2. Develops long lean muscles
3. Improves posture and alignment, which will relieve posture related disorders as well as improve general mobility so that one moves more fluidly and gracefully
4. Stimulates circulation and blood oxygenation as well as boosts immune system function
5. Improves mental clarity

Concentration

All movement originates in the mind. It is important to keep visualization and imagery active in physical movement. The more descriptive an instructor is in cueing a movement, the more he/she will bring the client into the moment and the better the performance of the movement.

Control

All physical movement is controlled by the mind. The more we involve the mind, the more we can eliminate excess or extraneous movement and produce the exact result intended.

Centering

All movements come from a stable center. Joseph Pilates called this center the Powerhouse. It should be compared to what we call the core in fitness. A good comparison would be the way a tree would function with a weak trunk and strong limbs. If the center isn't stable distal strength is useless. It is from a girdle of strength that one is stable and strong.

Breath

Pilates movements are coordinated with the breath. Inhalation brings in oxygen to feed the working phase and exhalation braces the core with the deep abdominals to maintain stability of the powerhouse.

Flow

Pilates exercises are performed gracefully, smoothly, and evenly. There is no use of momentum and there are no static exercises.

Precision

Concentrating on your movements and coordinating them with your breath improves kinesthetic awareness. Through Pilates exercise one learns how to use his or her body more effectively and efficiently.

Relaxation

Pilates exercises teach you to move without tension. They teach you to focus and concentrate.

Stamina

Pilates exercises improve the endurance of the muscles of the powerhouse. This allows for increased stability over long periods of time when performing everything from functional activities to sports.

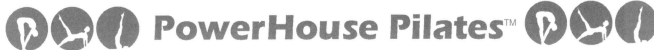

BREATHING

Breathing is an involuntary function over which we have limited control. For example, we can hold our breath temporarily, but the body will resume breathing on its own after enough oxygen is lost to cause unconsciousness. The body can use breath for relaxation or to increase metabolism. Heart rate and other basic body characteristics such as blood pressure are even affected by the rate or depth of the breath.

In pilates-based exercise, a full complete breath is used. The inhale is equal to the exhale in length. The inhale is taken through the nose and into the ribcage. It is helpful to think of the ribcage expanding east to west and the air going posteriorly. The exhale is through the mouth and there should be a sensation of hollowing in the abdomen as the diaphragm lifts to push all air from the lungs.

On the reformer a general rule is to inhale as your springs expand and exhale as they retract. Use the imagery of your ribcage expanding on the inhale.

There are many benefits to this breathing:

1. The inhale mobilizes the ribcage, improving posture of the upper body and decreasing the effects of normal aging on lung capacity.

2. The exhale engages the deep abdominal muscles including the transverse abdominis and the obliques that are vital for lumbar stability and protection of the lumbar spine in functional activities. This can also enhance the ability to call in the deep abdominal muscles effectively for exercise performance.

3. A complete breath increases relaxation by supplying oxygen to the working muscles and brain and releasing carbon dioxide from the body.

NEUTRAL SPINE

In all exercise based on the works of Joseph Pilates, the concept of a neutral spine is persistent. As the concept has been carried down, it has been described and cued in many different ways. It is truly the basis for good posture and effective use of the "Powerhouse".

In many explanations neutral spine and neutral pelvis are used interchangeably, but the two terms are not the same. Neutral pelvis is a component of neutral spine, when the pelvis lies in one plane. Neutral Spine is when all of the muscles of the body are balanced in length and strength, allowing the natural curves of the spine to exist: cervical lordosis, thoracic kyphosis, lumbar lordosis.

In the following list, you will find many different ways of arriving at the same neutral position. All are effective and correct methods of achieving neutral. Keep in mind that in a group setting it is important to have several methods or cues, so that you can communicate effectively. Some of the participants will respond to one cue, while others may need a different cue. A skilled instructor must be able to present the same concept in many different ways.

1) To find neutral pelvis, make your pubic symphysis and anterior superior iliac spines level to the floor.
2) Imagine your pelvis as a clock with your navel being 12, your pubis being 6, and each anterior superior iliac spine being 3 and 9 respectively. Neutral is half way between 12 and 6 and 3 and 9. Or, think of a pelvic bowl, and the water level and not swishing in any one direction.
3) Lie your tail bone on the floor and imagine a small grape in the small of your low back.
4) In the midback, imagine your ribcage parallel to the floor and all posterior rib surfaces touching the floor.
5) Reach long through the crown of your head, lengthening the back of your neck.

Remember that although we use neutral spine for many of the exercises, we do move in and out of neutral. It is this muscle memory that protects us as we move out of neutral, challenging spinal stability.

ANATOMY REVIEW

The roots of pilates based exercise are in efficient function of the musculoskeletal system. This function requires a balance of muscle length and strength not only in the limbs, but in what Joseph H. Pilates called the "Powerhouse" or the physical center. This area includes the entire trunk and encompasses the shoulder and pelvic girdles. With a thorough understanding of the pelvic and shoulder girdles an instructor will be able to effectively teach efficient movement and identify imbalance.

When you look closely at a girdle in the human body, you find a group of joints that work together. The shoulder girdle is made up of the manubrium (top part of the sternum) in the front, with a clavicle on each side leading to the scapulae in the back. The circle is completed by muscle connecting to the spine and ribcage. There are actually four shoulder joints on either side:

1) The sternoclavicular joint   3) The glenohumeral joint
2) The acromioclavicular joint   4) The scapulothoracic joint

These four joints work together to provide distal mobility and proximal stability in the upper body. There are many muscles involved in the efficient performance of the this girdle. The more noticeable ones are as follows:

1) Pectoralis Major/Minor   7) Sternocleido Mastoid
2) Rhomboids   8) Biceps
3) Trapezius   9) Triceps
4) Deltoid   10) Latissimus Dorsi
5) Rotator Cuff   11) Levator Scapula
6) Serratus Anterior

The second girdle involved in the Pilates powerhouse is the pelvic girdle. It is made up of the (ilium, ischium and pubis) hip bones, femur, sacrum and lumbar spine. The joints in the pelvic girdle are:

1) Sacroiliac joint
2) Lumbosacral joint
3) Pubic Symphysis
4) Hip joints

These joints work together to provide distal mobility and proximal stability in the lower body.

There are many muscles involved in the lower body and we will group many of them together according to their action:

1) Abdominals (Rectus Abdominis, Transverse Abdominis, Internal & External Obliques)
2) Back Extensors
3) Quadratus Lumborum
4) Hip Extensors (Gluteus Maximus and Minimus)
5) Hip Flexors (Iliopsoal, Rectus Femoris)
6) Hip Internal Rotators (Tensor Fascia Latae and Gluteus Minimus)
7) Hip External Rotators (Gluteus Maximus, Piriformis)
8) Hip Abductors (Tensor Fascia Latae and Gluteus Medius)
9) Hip Adductors

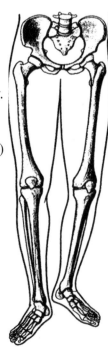

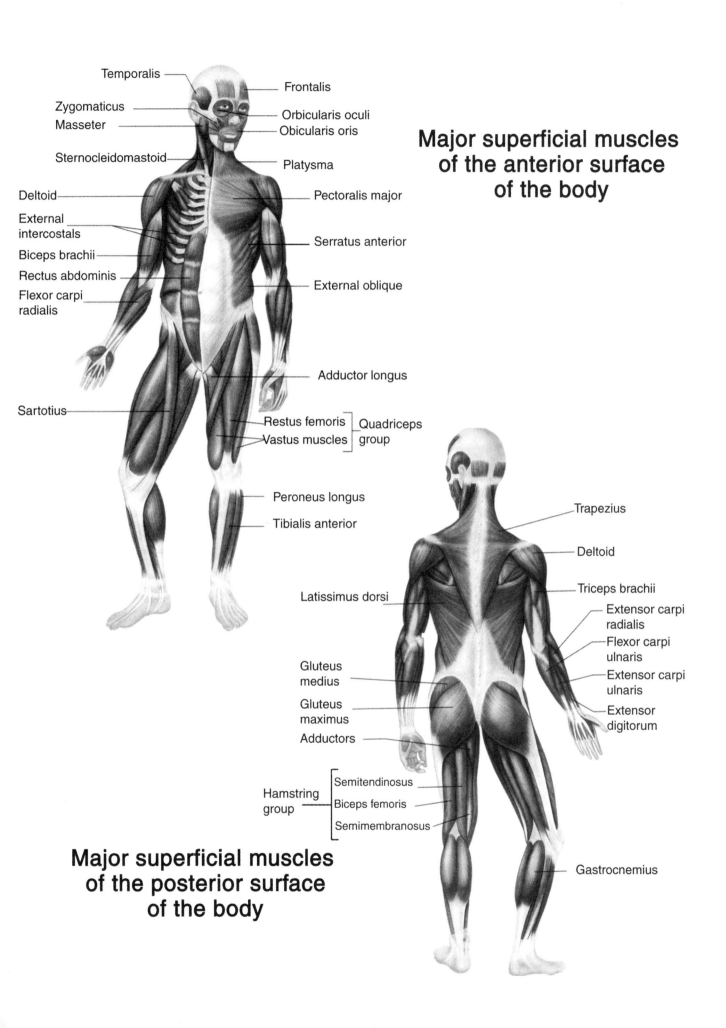

Temporalis

Frontalis

Zygomaticus

Orbicularis oculi

Masseter

Obicularis oris

Sternocleidomastoid

Platysma

Deltoid

Pectoralis major

External intercostals

Serratus anterior

Biceps brachii

Rectus abdominis

Flexor carpi radialis

External oblique

Adductor longus

Sartotius

Restus femoris   Quadriceps
Vastus muscles   group

Peroneus longus

Tibialis anterior

Major superficial muscles
of the anterior surface
of the body

Trapezius

Deltoid

Triceps brachii

Latissimus dorsi

Extensor carpi
radialis

Flexor carpi
ulnaris

Extensor carpi
ulnaris

Extensor
digitorum

Gluteus
medius

Gluteus
maximus

Adductors

Semitendinosus

Hamstring
group

Biceps femoris

Semimembranosus

Gastrocnemius

Major superficial muscles
of the posterior surface
of the body

COMMON POSTURES

Lordotic - This posture is what we call "the cheerleader." Characteristics include an increase in the normal lumbar lordosis, a sacral inclination, and an anterior pelvic tilt. With this posture you will often find tightness in the hip flexors, erector spinae, and/or internal rotators of the hip. There will be weakness of the hamstrings, abdominals, and/or external rotators of the hip. This posture in the lower spine often causes a compensatory increase in the cervical lordosis with tightness in the suboccipital muscles.

Flat Back - This posture is what we call "the guy," as it is a common male posture. Characteristics include a decrease in the lumbar lordosis and a posterior pelvic tilt. With this posture you will often find tightness of the hamstrings and external rotators of the hip. There will be weakness in the lumbar erector spinae and in the hip internal rotators. This posture often causes a compensatory flattened cervical curve with tightness in the neck flexors. Participants with this posture are rigid and lack mobility of the torso.

Kyphotic - In this posture the muscles of the upper back are lengthened and the muscles of the chest are shortened with a collapsing of the chest. The head is forward and the neck flexors and suboccipitals are short. The pelvis is generally posterior tilted or neutral. This posture can inhibit respiration and the breathing in Pilates-based exercise can improve it drastically by mobilization of the rib cage.

Sway Back - In this posture the pelvis is posterior tilted but also pushed forward in the sagittal plane. The rib cage is collapsed and for balance the trunk is shifted backward in the sagittal plane. Hamstrings are shortened and hip flexors are lengthened. Shoulders are rounded with tight chest muscles and neck flexors.

Forward Head - This is often a compensatory posture to the above postures due to the effect of gravity on the spine. The muscles involved are the levator scapulae, upper trapezius, sternocleidomastoid, scalene, and suboccipital muscles. This posture occurs when the neck flexors become tight and strong and the long extensors become lengthened and weak. This orients the gaze downward and the head forward of the shoulders. To correct the gaze and balance, the suboccipital muscles contract holding the head in a level position.

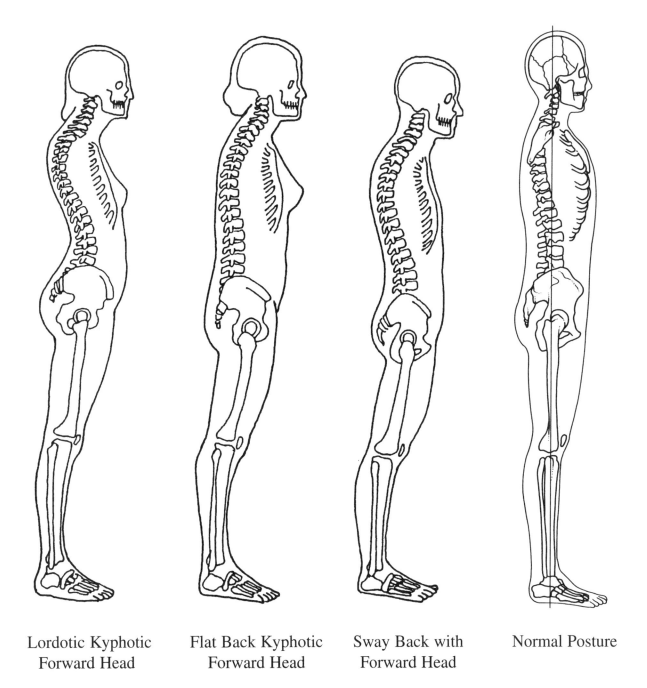

Lordotic Kyphotic
Forward Head

Flat Back Kyphotic
Forward Head

Sway Back with
Forward Head

Normal Posture

NORMAL STATIC POSTURE

For a weight-bearing joint to be stable there must be a force to counteract the force of gravity. In the body the counter force is either muscle/tendon or ligament/tissue. Evaluating clients' posture is the key to designing a program to meet their needs. Think of a posture as window to imbalance. When you identify the posture you can assume the tight and weak muscles. Begin by getting an overall visual scan of the client.

Lateral Plumb Line Posture—View the client from the side and imagine a plumb line running from the ceiling to the floor. The plumb line should pass through the following points in good static posture:
1. **Mastoid Process**—bony prominence just behind the ear.
   - The center of gravity of the head is in front of the head to neck junction (atlanto-occipital joints). The muscles in the back of the neck contract to balance the head.
2. A point just in front of the **glenohumeral joint** (largest shoulder joint).
   - In the trunk, the gravity line goes through the bodies of the lumbar and cervical vertebrae. This balances the spinal curves. There is activity of the erector spinae to maintain balance.
3. The **hip joints** (or just behind).
   - When the gravity line passes through the hip there is equilibrium.
   - When the gravity line passes behind the hip it causes a posterior tilt of the pelvis (the "guy" posture) and is controlled by the tension of the hip flexors.
4. A point just in front of the center of the **knee joints**.
   - Keeps the knee in extension and therefore requires no muscle support
   - Stability is provided by the ligaments and capsule of the knee and by the posterior muscles, including the gastrocnemius and the hamstrings
   - If the knees flex, the gravity line shifts posteriorly and the quadriceps must contract to keep the knees from buckling.
5. A point just in front of the **ankle joints**.
   - The plantar flexor muscles, primarily the soleus, provide stability.

Posterior View- View the client from the back looking for asymmetry or gross deformity.
1. Head and neck- should be straight with no tilt to either side.
2. Shoulders- should be even in height, although the dominant side is often lower. The scapulae should be flat on the back (no winging) and their medial borders should be equal distance from the thoracic spine.
3. Iliac crests- should be even in height.
4. Sacral iliac joints- should be even in height.
5. Gluteal folds- should be even in height.
6. Knee folds- should be even in height.
7. Feet and ankles- look for asymmetry as well as supination or pronation in the foot or varus and valgus in the ankle.
8. Muscle balance- Look for asymmetry of muscle bellies. Watch for atrophy of one side.
9. Spine- Look for gross abnormalities such as scoliosis, rotoscoliosis, or extreme thoracic kyphosis.

It is beneficial to make general notes on your observation of the client to assist with program planning and to evaluate progress. Avoid sharing much of this information with the client or diagnosing him or her in any way. This assessment is subjective and is meant only to assist the teacher in designing a personal training program.

COMMON PROBLEMS

Please note that these are not diagnoses of conditions, only a possible cause of the imbalance that a participant may be experiencing. Use these problems to help you understand what modifications of the exercises that might help a participant. Make sure when tailoring a workout specifically for a client that it is a balanced complete overall body workout and only targets certain areas briefly.

Winging shoulder blades—Possible cause: Weakness in back muscles.
Have participants protract their shoulder blades and hold this position while weight bearing. Do not challenge participants into more advanced exercises until they can maintain scapula stability.

"Boinking" ribcage—Possible cause: Weakness in abdominal muscles.
Try to have a participant maintain neutral pelvic alignment for less challenging exercises, even if the ribcage is not in line with the pelvis. Raising the headrest can often help to keep the ribcage down. For more advanced exercises, place the pelvis in a posterior tilt and maintain ribcage-pelvic alignment.

Inability to open chest—Possible cause: Tightness in chest muscles.
Work on exercises that strengthen the back muscles and stretch the chest muscles. Take care to work the body in balanced manner.

Inability to long sit—Possible cause: Tightness in hamstrings.
Encourage clients to do exercises to stretch the hamstrings, like Elephant. However until they can maintain neutral alignment while in this position, have them sit cross-legged during all seated exercises.

Painful Wrists—Possible cause: Weakness in wrist area.
Modify the exercise to have less weight in the hands. However, encourage weight bearing for as long as they can to strengthen the hands and forearms.

Painful neck—Possible causes: Weakness in abdominal muscles.
Usually as participants abdominal muscles get stronger they will be able to maintain a more comfortable position with their head when lifted. Have them put their head back onto the carriage when their neck becomes fatigued.

Soreness in the hip flexor area—Possible cause: Tightness in hip flexor muscles or hamstrings.
Allow participants time to stretch between exercises that cause discomfort. Work on creating muscle balance with exercises that specifically target the hip flexor area (Eve's Lunge); and the hamstring area (Elephant) If this happens in a seated position, sit cross legged or bowl sit with the hips in external rotation.

Fatigue or pain on leg circles—Possible cause: Hip muscle imbalance.
Allow participants to bend their knees if their hamstrings are very tight, keeping the thigh at a 90° angle with the hip. All movement should initiate from the hip. As their hamstrings become more flexible they will have less discomfort. Beginners should rest in between if they become fatigued and cannot maintain form.

Stabilization

An area of the body is stable or has stability when it is able to maintain a neutral static posture while performing a desired activity. The static posture is maintained by a balance in length and strength of opposing large muscle groups and by a balanced static muscle tension of smaller deep muscle groups. At times the loss of stability is due to an improper focus of the participant. It could be a learned pattern, or just an inability or lack of understanding of how to move the body in space.

There are three main areas of the body that will require stability to perform the Pilates program effectively.
Pelvic Stability –the ability to hold the pelvis in a neutral position, while using the lower extremities or upper torso.

> **Neutral Pelvis**- A position halfway between a forward tilt of the pelvis and a backward tilt of the pelvis, where the muscles about the pelvis can function with even strength and length for long periods of time. For most individuals, this will be when the ASIS'S and the pubic symphysis are in the frontal plane. There will be a natural lordosis present.
>
> **What causes one to lose pelvic stability?** Pelvic stability is lost when the intrinsic muscles are not strong enough to fight the pull of the larger working muscle or when there is an imbalance between opposing large muscle groups.

Torso Stability – the ability to maintain the torso position while working the limbs.

> **Neutral Spine** –Involves all curves of the spine. A position where there is equal tension of anterior and posterior muscles, allowing for muscle balance in the spine and pelvis so that the natural spinal curves can be maintained.
>
> **What causes one to lose torso stability?** Muscle imbalance or weakness of intrinsic muscles will cause loss of stability.

Scapular Stability – the ability to hold the shoulder girdle in neutral while using the upper extremities.

> **Neutral Shoulder Girdle**- A position where there is balanced tension of intrinsic and extrinsic muscles of the shoulder to allow efficient alignment of the shoulder joints for optimum function.
>
> **What causes us to lose scapular stability?** Muscle imbalance or weakness of intrinsic muscles will cause loss of stability.

Neutral spine described by body position:

Supine – Pelvic neutral + ribcage neutral + cervical neutral= neutral spine
In this position the muscles should be at rest when you are lying on the floor. Note that many will feel uncomfortable in this position as they have imbalances of length and strength in the torso.

Prone – To find neutral alignment in the prone position, place the ASIS's and pubic symphysis again in the frontal plane. If the arms are overhead, draw the anterior portion of the 10th rib into the same frontal plane. Reach long through the crown of your head and avoid cervical hyperextension. To protect the spine in back extension, keep the pubic symphysis on the floor and/or in line with the ASIS's. As you perform exercises that move the extremities or spine use the "Principle of Extension"– lengthen the spine as you extend.

Sidelying – To find neutral stack the hips and reach long with the top leg to create a small unweighted area at your waist.

Plank - To find neutral alignment in the plank position, the ASIS and pubic symphysis should be in the frontal plane of the body (actually at a slight angle to the floor). The coccyx will point between the legs and the shoulder blades will be down and flat on the back. An unstable shoulder (one with muscle imbalance) will show winging shoulder blades. An imbalance in the pelvic area will show a sagging or lifted middle.

Seated- To find neutral alignment in the seated position, the sits bones need to be on the floor with the ASIS and pubic symphysis in the frontal plane. The shoulders should be down and back with the neck long and the head over the shoulders.

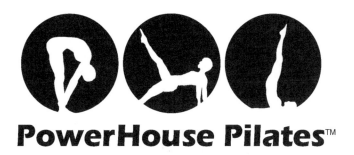

PowerHouse Pilates™

BEGINNER
REFORMER EXERCISES

This section is designed to help you get started teaching basic Pilates Reformer exercises to your clientele. As a beginning Pilates instructor, mastering these exercises using the Pilates principles will help you to understand how to adapt and modify as you progress to more advanced exercises.

Use this selection of exercises to design your beginning group reformer classes. Always remember to be aware of the variations in each exercise to help you modify the exercises for your novice clientele. Keep your number of repetitions low in the beginning and slowly progress your clients to ensure success of your Pilates Reformer program. Most of all have fun with your classes! Make Pilates exercise fun and rewarding.

Contrology® develops the body uniformly, corrects wrong postures, restores physical vitality, invigorates the mind and elevates the spirit.

Joseph H. Pilates

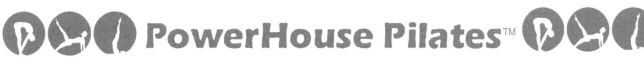
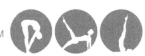

FOOTWORK

Category: Warm up, cool down

Benefits: Heat builder, flexibility and strengthening of the lower body, awareness of spinal neutral, breath with movement, proximal stability and distal mobility.

Breathing: Inhale as you move the carriage back and exhale as you return home.

Repetitions: 8 to 10

Springs: 3 to 4   PETIT   2 RED, 1 BLUE
                      NORMAL HT - 3 RED

Prerequisites: The ability to maintain neutral during movement.

Footwork I Movement: Push the carriage back without locking the knees, drop the heels under the bar, toe raise and then return home.

Variations: Do the same with the balls of the feet on the bar and the heels in line with the ischial tuberosities, or with the balls of the feet on the bar and feet touching together. Do the movement as a combination or split the calf raise and leg press sections.

Footwork II Movement: Push the carriage back without locking the knees and then return home.

- FOOTBAR IN HIGH POSITION
- INHALE PUSH BACK
- EXHALE DRAW UP
- RESIST & DRAW FORWARD

VARIATIONS: 2 RED / BICYCLE

RT LEG TABLE TOP
PUSHBACK - COME HOME & ST. LEG OVER BAR

Cues:

- Keep the knees over the second toes.
- Keep the knees from turning in (femoral anteversion) when pressing back.
- Zip the inner thighs together as you press back.
- Feel a wrapping sensation in the buttocks.
- Widen the back and soften the neck.
- Reach the knees to the ceiling as you return the carriage home.

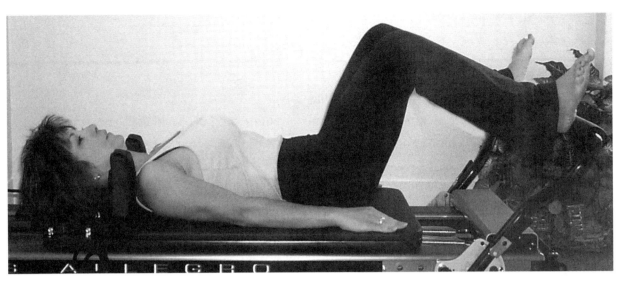

Footwork Set Up

Pilates V and Parallel Set Up: Lie supine on the carriage with the head rest up. Place your pelvis and rib cage in neutral. Place the balls of the feet on the footbar with the toes curled softly over. Place your feet either in "Pilates V" by turning out at the hips or align your heels with your ischial tuberosities for a parallel position. *RELAX HEELS*

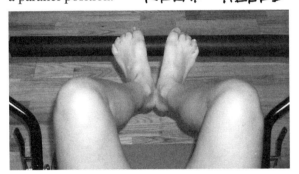

Pilates V

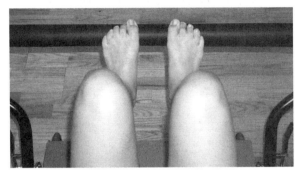

Balls Of Feet Parallel

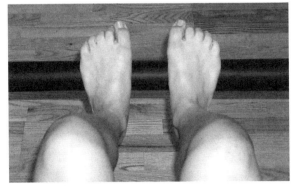

Bird On A Perch

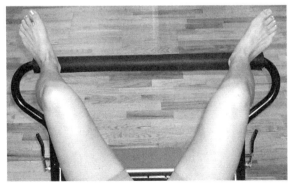

Heels On

Bird on a Perch Set Up: Lie supine on the carriage with the head rest up and the pelvis and ribcage in neutral. Place the heads of the metatarsals on the footbar with the toes curled softly over and heels in line with the ischial tuberosities.

Heels On Set Up: Lie supine on the carraige with the heels on the footbar at ischial tuberisities and the feet flexed, hips in external rotation and abducted wider than the shoulders. Keep the knees over the second toes.

25

PELVIC LIFT

HEADSET DOWN

Category: Core stability, lower body strengthening.

Benefits: Heat builder, flexibility of the spine, strengthening of the gluteus maximus, awareness of spinal neutral during movement, breath with movement, proximal stability and distal mobility.

Breathing: Inhale as you move the carriage back and exhale as you return home.

Variations: Have participants do the pelvic lift and spinal articulation without moving the carriage back to learn to use the deep abdominals.

Prerequisites: Bridging on the mat with spinal articulation.

Repetitions: 8 to 10

Springs: 3 to 4   2 R , 1B or 3R ; 2 RED / MORE ADVANCED

- INHALE TO STAY
- EXHALE TO BRIDGE : PEEL UP
- INHALE - PUSH BACK
- EXHALE - RETURN HOME

Cues:
- Keep the knees over the second toes.
- Keep ribcage and pelvis aligned throughout the exercise.
- Stay on your shoulder blades as you complete the movement.
- Stay off of your neck.
- Keep your shoulders down and your back wide.

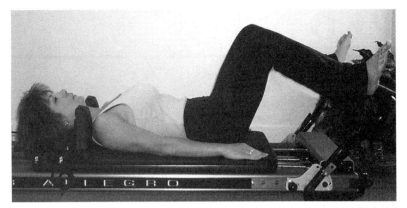

Set Up: Lie supine on the carriage with the head rest down and the pelvis and ribcage in neutral. Arms are flat on the carriage. Place the heels of the feet on the outside of the footbar with the feet flexed and knees over the second toe.

CAN DO W/ FEET PARALLEL

Pelvic Lift Set Up

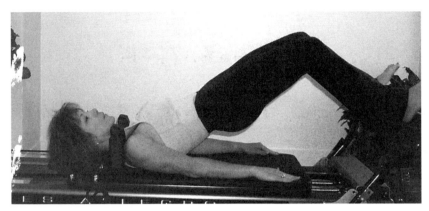

Pelvic Lift Articulating Bridge

Movement: Begin by tilting pubic bone toward the ceiling and articulating the spine off the carriage one vertebrae at a time until you are on your shoulders blades. Hold this position as you push the carriage back and forth with your legs.

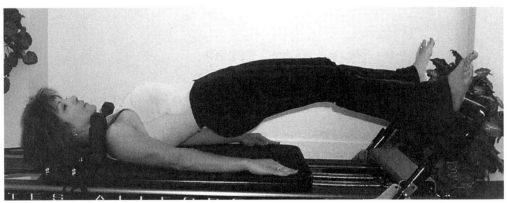

Pelvic Lift Movement

·KEEP CARRAIGE STILL
·IF CAN'T HOLD LEGS IN TABLETOP, PUT FEET ON BAR

THE HUNDRED

Category: Warm up, core stability.

Benefits: Heat builder, strengthening of the deep abdominals and neck, lumbar flexibility breath with movement, proximal stability and distal mobility.

Set Up: Lie supine on the carriage with the pelvis and ribcage in neutral and hips and knees flexed to 90 degrees. Hands hold the small loops with elbows on the carriage and palms facing the footbar. CAN DO HEADREST UP

Breathing: Inhale for 5 slaps and exhale for 5 slaps. To increase difficulty think of pumping up a tire on the inhale and pausing deflation on the exhale.

Prerequisites: Hundreds on the mat.

Repetitions: 10 sets of 10

Springs: 1 to 2   1 R ; 1 R, 1 B OR 1 R, 1 Y, 2 R

· INHALE TO STAY
· EXHALE - ROLL UP AS U ROLL HEAD & SHOULDERS OFF
· REACH LONG THRU STRAPS w/ ARMS
· KEEP CARRIAGE STILL AS SPLASH H₂0

Cues: PRESS INTO STRAPS
- Keep a wide broad back.
- Reach through your arms and keep them low to the carriage.
- Squeeze knees and ankles together.
- Keep your sacrum on the carriage.
- Drop navel to spine on the exhale and inhale into the back of the ribcage.
- Hold the pelvis in neutral as you flex the spine.

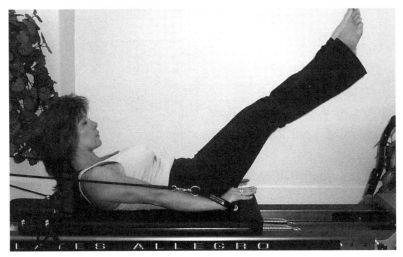
Hundred Movement

Movement: Raise the head and shoulders rounding the spine as you reach the hands toward the footbar by extending the elbows. Begin to move your arms from the shoulder joint only, as if you were slapping water. Inhale and exhale while keeping the carriage still after the head and shoulders are lifted.

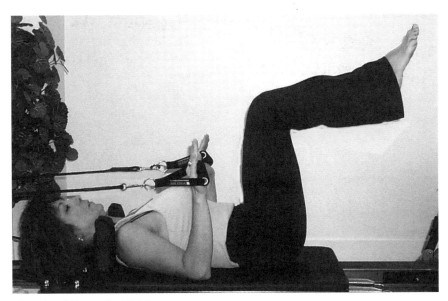
Hundred Legs In Tabletop

Variations: To decrease difficulty, place the legs in tabletop position. Extend the hips and knees in "Pilates V" to increase difficulty. Leave the feet on the footbar or head on headrest to decrease difficulty. Begin with arms extended straight to the ceiling and do shoulder extension as you raise your head to increase difficulty.

COORDINATION

Category: Core strengthening and stability, lower body strengthening.

Benefits: Strengthening of the powerhouse and lower body, breath with movement, proximal stability and distal mobility.

Breathing: Exhale, as you raise your head and shoulders and extend your arms and legs. Inhale as you open and close your legs, exhale as you draw your hips and knees and then your elbows into flexion.

Variations: To lessen the difficulty, break the exercise into parts. Keep the lower extremities flexed, or the head and shoulders on the carriage. To increase the difficulty add 5 leg crosses and 5 heel beats in "Pilates V" on the last repetition.

Prerequisites: Coordination or Hundreds on the mat.

Repetitions: 8 to 10   2-3 SETS   START W/ ARMS EXT OR KNEES BENT

Springs: 1 to 2   I R   SAME RESISTANCE AS 100's

- START IN 100's POSITION
- OPEN LEGS
- OPEN & CLOSE
- BRING TO GETHER
- DROP LEG TO TABLETOP

(DON'T BRING HEAD & shd BACK DWN WHEN BRING KNEES IN

Cues:
- Reach through the arms and widen the back.
- Look toward your thighs and keep your chin off your chest.
- Do not allow your torso or pelvis to rock back and forth.

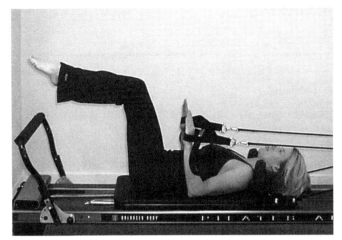

Coordination Set Up

Set Up: Lie supine on the carriage with the pelvis and ribcage in neutral. Your hips and knees are flexed to 90 degrees. Hands hold the small loops with elbows on the carriage and palms facing the footbar.

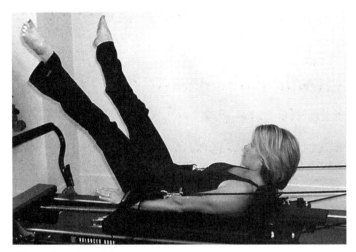

Coordination Movement

Movement: Raise the head and shoulders rounding the spine as you reach the hands toward the footbar and extend the elbows. At the same time extend the lower extremities between 90 and 45 degrees in "Pilates V". Hold this position as you abduct and adduct the hips to shoulder width one time. With the head and shoulders still elevated, bring the lower extremities back to 90 degrees of hip and knee flexion and then the elbows to 90 degrees of flexion. Continue to keep the head and shoulders elevated as you perform the recommended repetitions and on the last repetition allow them to return to neutral.

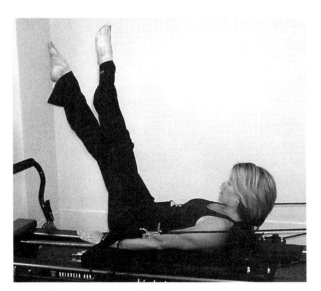

Coordination Leg Crosses

31

- DON'T RAISE HANDS ABOVE ShDs
  (PAST)
- KEEP ShD BLADES DRAWN DOWN BACK WHILE CIRCLING
- WATCH FOR RIBCAGE LIFTING WHILE CIRCLING

ARM CIRCLES

Category: Upper body strengthening, core stability.

Benefits: Strengthening of the upper body, awareness of spinal neutral, breath with movement, proximal stability and distal mobility.

Breathing: Inhale as your springs expand and exhale as they retract.

Variations: To lessen the difficulty, break the motions down and do them in pieces. For limited or painful shoulder motion, do the circle with your elbows resting on the carriage and flexed to 90 degrees.

Prerequisites: Arm circles on the mat while maintaining neutral.

Repetitions: 8 to 10

Springs: 1 to 2   1 R, 1 B ; 1 R + 1 Y IF STRONGER

- HEADREST UP
- MAINTAIN TABLETOP - SQUEEZE KNEES
- ARMS IN FRONT OF ShDs
- INHALE - BRING ARMS ↓
- EXHALE TO BRING ARMS UP

Cues:
- Maintain neutral at the ribcage and the pelvis.
- Soften the neck.
- Squeeze the knees and ankles together.
- Lengthen and reach through your arms as you circle.
- Make sure not to circle your arms above the shoulder rests.

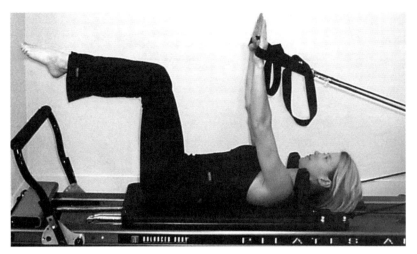

Arm Circles Set Up

Set Up: Lie supine on the carriage with the pelvis and ribcage in neutral. Hips and knees are flexed at 90 degrees. Place hands in the small loops and adjust the length so that the carriage is floating when the arms are extended to the ceiling at a level lower than the shoulder rests.

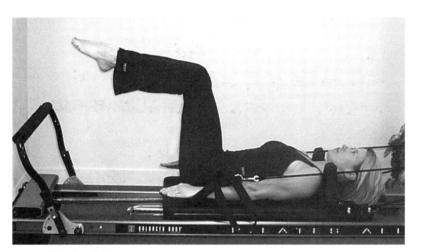

Arm Circles Movement

Movement: Draw the arms down to the carriage, turn palms slightly to the ceiling as you raise the arms in abduction and then horizontally adduct to the starting position. To reverse the circle, open the arms in horizontal abduction, adduct to sides and then forward flex to the starting position.

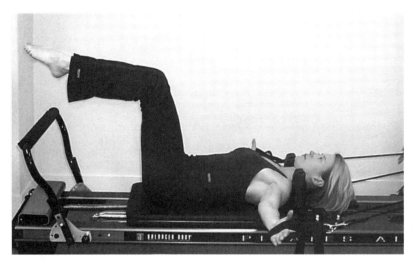

Arm Circles Movement

33

- SACRUM ON CARRIAGE
- BEND LEGS IN 1ST
- WRAP & ZIP LEGS

LEG CIRCLES

Category: Lower body strengthening, core stability.

Benefits: Strengthening of the lower body, awareness of spinal neutral, breath with movement, proximal stability and distal mobility, hip range of motion or flexibility.

Breathing: Inhale as you move the carriage back and exhale as you return home.

Variations: To decrease the difficulty, move the strap to below the knee and do the movement with a bent leg.

Prerequisites: Leg circles on the mat.

Repetitions: 8 to 10

Springs: 2 to 3   SAME AS FOOT WORK
          PETIT   2 R; 1 Y

- BUTT ON CARRIAGE
- INHALE ↓ ; EXHALE CIRCLE OUT & AROUND
- INHALE OPEN ; EXHALE BACK TO START

SPLIT - INHALE OPEN
        EXHALE PULL TOGETHER
        KEEP P. V - CARRIAGE WILL MOVE W/ U

Cues:
- Keep the sacrum on the carriage at all times.
- Zip the inner thighs together when performing adduction.
- Feel a wrapping sensation in the buttocks.
- Widen the back and soften the neck.
- Reach your toes for the walls and lengthen through your legs.

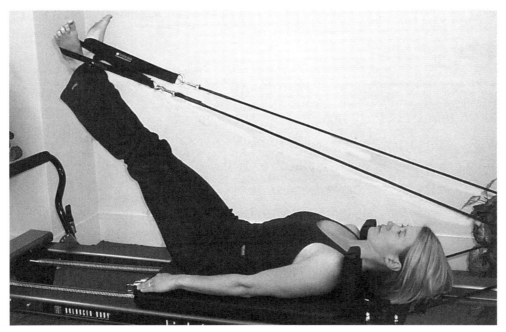

Leg Circles Set Up

Set Up: Lie supine on the carriage with pelvis and ribcage in neutral. Place the long arches of the feet in the large loops with the knees softly extended and the hips as close to 90 degrees as possible.

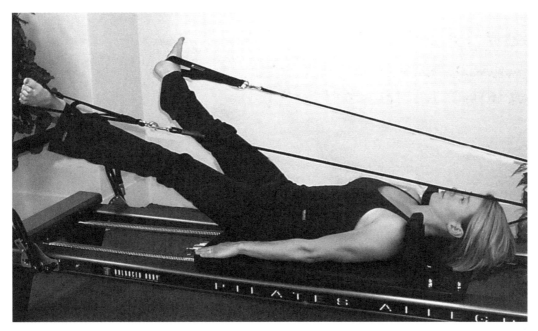

Leg Circles Movement

Movement: Extend the lower extremities toward the carriage as a unit without losing pelvic neutral. Abduct and externally rotate the hips as you move through hip flexion to return to the starting position. To reverse the circle, abduct the hips and then extend and adduct the hips as you push the carriage back. Bring the legs together as you perform hip flexion to return to the starting position. Be sure to remain in spinal neutral.

FROG

Category: Lower extremity strengthening, core stability.

Benefits: Flexibility and strengthening of the lower body, awareness of spinal neutral, breath with movement, proximal stability and distal mobility.

Breathing: Inhale as you move the carriage back and exhale as you return home.

Variations: To decrease the difficulty, keep the lower extremities near 90 degrees of hip flexion as they extend. To increase difficulty, keep the lower extremities closer to 45 degrees of hip flexion or lower. To increase flexibility and improve coordination, try this exercise as a single leg with the other leg riding along in either an abducted or flexed position.

Prerequisites: The ability to maintain neutral and "Pilates V" with legs extended from your body on the mat.

Repetitions: 8 to 10

Springs: 2 to 3 R

- INHALE AS U DRAW HEELS TO BUTT
- EXHALE TO PUSH AWAY ; WRAP

SINGLE LEG FROG:
- INHALE AS DRAW LEG IN
- EXHALE AS PUSH AWAY

Cues:
- Keep the knees over the second toes.
- Keep the heels together throughout the movement.
- Zip the inner thighs together as you press back.
- Feel a wrapping sensation in the buttocks.
- Widen the back and soften the neck.

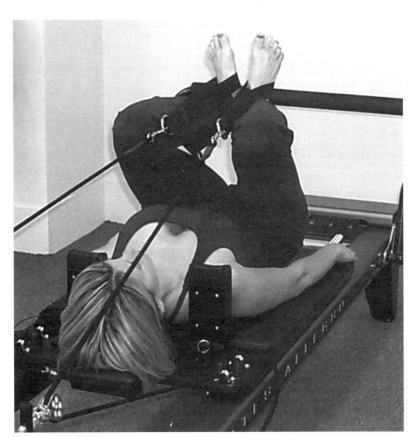

Frog Set Up

Set Up: Lie supine on the carriage with the pelvis and ribcage in neutral and the large loops around the long arches of the feet. The lower extremities are extended between 90 and 45 degrees of flexion in "Pilates V".

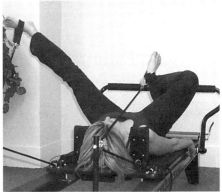

Frog Single Leg

Movement: Draw your heels toward your buttocks while maintaining pelvic neutral and then extend knees and hips outward along the same line. Act as though your heels were drawing a line and retracing it over and over.

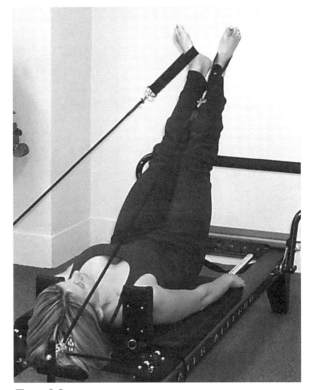

Frog Movement

37

- KEEP HEADREST ↓

- HEAVIER WEIGHT HELPS PUT LEGS UP BUT TAKES MORE BACK TO PULL ↓

SHORT SPINE

Category: Core strengthening and flexibility.

Benefits: Flexibility and strengthening of the core and lower body, breath with movement.

Breathing: Inhale, and then exhale as you bring the feet over head and peel the spine from the carriage. Inhale as you bring your knees to the shoulder rests and press the spine into the carriage. Draw your feet to your seat and then exhale as you press out into frog.

Variations: For a better spine stretch keep the heels at the buttocks during the return to carriage phase. Try reversing the breathing to change the abdominal emphasis. Heavier springs will assist beginners. Shortening the straps by putting the feet in the small loops will increase the stretch.

Prerequisites: Frog on the reformer, rolling like a ball and spine stretch.

Repetitions: 8 to 10

Springs: 2 to 4 *2R, 1 B or Y*

Cues:
- Keep the knees over the second toe.
- Zip the inner thighs together as you press out into frog.
- Stop at the shoulder blades and do not roll onto the neck.
- Keep space between your ribcage and your pelvis.
- Keep your shoulders down and open in front.

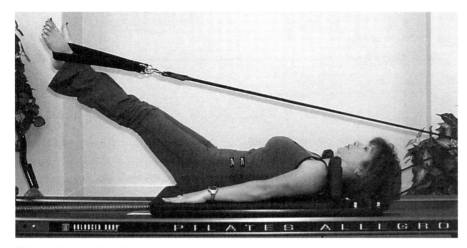

Short Spine Set Up

Set Up: Lie supine on the carriage with the head rest down, the feet in the small loops, and the lower extremities extended into "Pilates V". Pelvis and spine are in neutral with the <u>sacrum</u> on the <u>carriage</u>. The carriage will be in the pushed back position.

STRENGTHENS ABS &
LENGTHENS SPINE
BODY IN LETTER "J"

Movement: Allow the carriage to return home in a controlled manner as the spine peels from sacrum to shoulder blades, and the lower extremities extend over the head. When a full shoulder blade stand is reached, bring the knees toward the shoulder rests with the feet in "Pilates V". Maintaining a rounded position, roll the spine into the carriage one vertebrae at a time. When the sacrum is in contact, finish by pressing the lower extremities out in "Pilates V" as you would in frog.

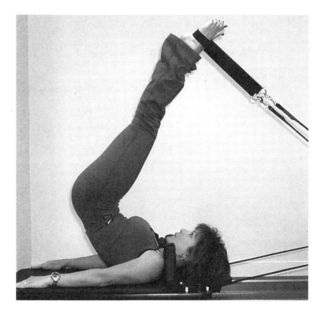

Short Spine Movement

BRING KNEES to SHD
RESTS; KEEP KNEES IN
LINE W/ 2ND TOE
. DON'T LET CARRIAGE
MOVE WHILE ROLLING

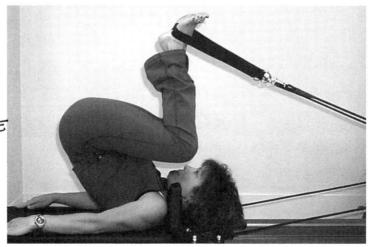

Short Spine Movement

39

DOWN STRETCH

Category: Core stability, upper body strengthening.

Benefits: Core stability, flexibility of the lower body, strengthening of the upper body, awareness of spinal neutral, breath with movement, proximal stability and distal mobility.

Breathing: Inhale as you move the carriage back and exhale as you return home.

Variations: Use two springs to feel more arm work and one spring to feel more core work.

Prerequisites: The ability to perform a modified push up on your knees while maintaining neutral spine.

Repetitions: 8 to 10

Springs: 1 to 2   1R

- HANDS ARE WIDE
- TO STOP WINGING VISUALIZE ICE CUBES UNDER ARMPITS

Cues:
- Widen the back and reach out through the crown of your head.
- Do not allow the scapulae to wing.
- Move in a half moon or crescent line.
- Imagine lying the front of your thighs on the carriage as you push back.

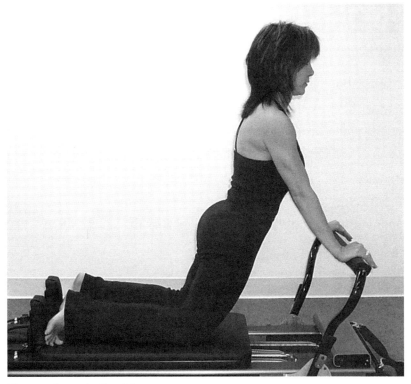

Set Up: Kneel on the carriage with your heels in line with your ischial tuberosities and your feet against the shoulder rests. Drop your anterior iliac spine (ASIS) toward the footbar and aim your tail bone between your legs. Elbows are extended and thumbs are in line with your fingers.

Down Stretch Set Up

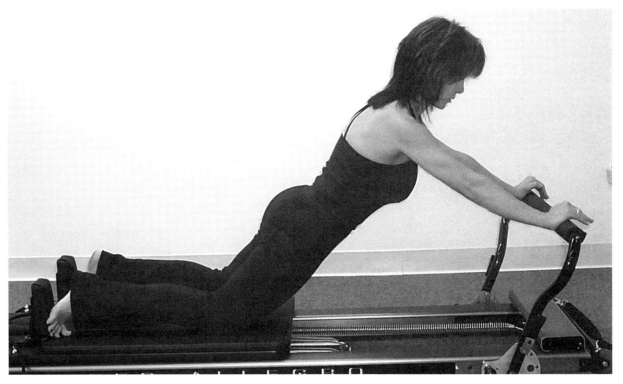

Down Stretch Movement

Movement: Push the carriage back without loosing your spinal position. Return the carriage reaching out through the crown of your head. Elbows stay extended.

LONG STRETCH

Category: Upper body strengthening, core stability.

Benefits: Strengthening of the upper body, scapular stability, awareness of spinal neutral, breath with movement, proximal stability and distal mobility.

Breathing: Inhale as you move the carriage back and exhale as you return home.

Variations: To increase the difficulty, reduce to one spring, bring feet closer together at the headrest, or move the carriage further back.

Prerequisites: Plank on the mat without shoulders "winging" or loss of neutral spine.

Repetitions: 8 to 10   (3~4)

Springs: 1 to 2

- INHALE PUSH BACK
- EXHALE UP & OVER

Cues:

- Press into the hands and widen the back for scapular stability.
- Reach long through the crown of your head.
- Keep the thumbs in line with the fingers and do not grip the bar.
- Avoid hyperextension of the elbows.

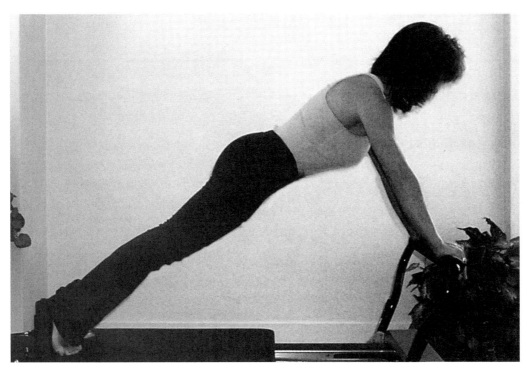

Long Stretch Set Up

Set Up: Get into a plank position with your hands on the footbar and your feet in front of the shoulder rests. Rest on the balls of the feet with your heels against the shoulder rests. Take the spine and pelvis to neutral and widen the back.

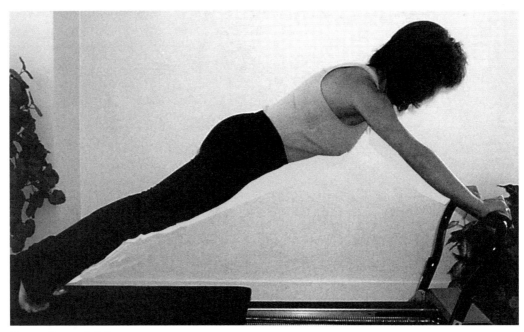

Long Stretch Movement

Movement: Push the carriage back with straight elbows while maintaining neutral spine and then return the carriage bringing the face over the footbar.

MOVE FOOT BAR ↑ 1 NOTCH

ELEPHANT

Category: Core strengthening, lower body flexibility, upper body strengthening.

Benefits: Flexibility and strengthening of the calves and hamstrings, strengthening of the deep abdominals, shoulder stability, thoracic extension, breath with movement, proximal stability and distal mobility.

Breathing: Inhale as you move the carriage back and exhale as you return home.

Variations: To increase the stretch, try raising the toes off of the carriage. To relieve the stretch bend the knees slightly. Try this exercise with a round back.

Prerequisites: "Down dog" position on the mat comfortably without losing spinal neutral.

Repetitions: 8 to 10

Springs: 2 to 3   1 B + 1 R   OR   1 R + 1 Y

- PUT SITS BONES BEHIND HEELS
- INHALE - PUSH BACK
- EXHALE COME IN
- PUSH UP TOES FOR CALF STRETCH
- NAVEL TO SPINE TO PULL LEGS UNDER

Cues:
- Keep the ischial tuberosities to the ceiling.
- Think of your body as an upside down V.
- Draw the navel to the spine as you bring the carriage home.
- Keep your upper body stable and hinge only from the hips.
- Maintain a small range of motion.

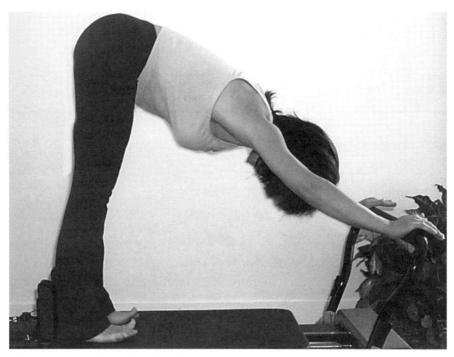

Elephant Set Up (Flat Back)

Set Up: Stand on the carriage with your heels in front of the shoulder rests and your hands shoulder width apart on the footbar. Point your ischial tuberosities toward the ceiling and press your chest toward your thighs. Put your ears between your elbows and look to your thighs.

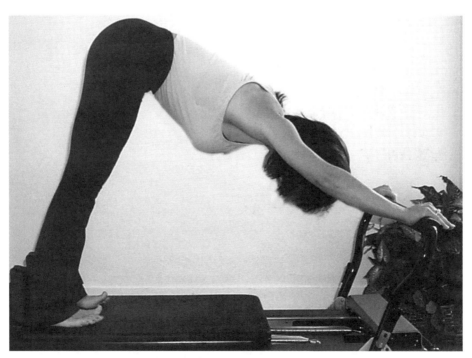

Elephant Movement (Flat Back)

Movement: Push the carriage back using only the lower the extremities moving only at the hip joint. Return the carriage with control using the deep abdominals.

45

STOMACH MASSAGE
Round Back

Category: Core stability, lower body flexibility and strengthening.

Benefits: Flexibility and strengthening of the lower body, spinal flexion, breath with movement, proximal stability and distal mobility.

Breathing: Inhale as you move the carriage back and exhale as you return home.

Variations: To decrease difficulty, break up the motions of pushing back and calf raising into small segments. As an added stretch for cool down, grasp the footbar with your hands and turn feet to parallel. Then glide the carriage back extending the knees for a hamstring and low back stretch.

Prerequisites: Spine stretch on the mat.

Repetitions: 5 to 8

Springs: 1 to 2

INHALE PUSH OUT
EXHALE COME IN

LOWER FT BAR ↓

Cues:
- Keep the knees over the second toes.
- Zip the inner thighs together as you press back.
- Keep shoulders directly over the hips throughout the movement.
- Stay on ischial tuberosities throughout exercise.
- Keep a small space between your chin and chest
- Lengthen your spine as you flex forward.

46

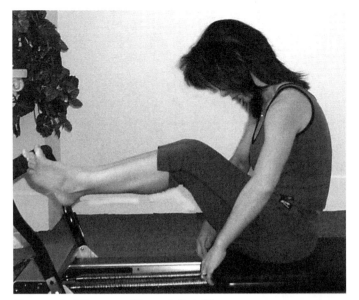

Stomach Massage Round Set Up

Set Up: Sit on the carriage with your feet in "Pilates V" and balls of the feet on the footbar. Sit as close to the footbar as you can and round your back into a "C" curve. Align your shoulders directly above your hips. Curl your fingers around the front edge of the carriage.

Movement: While maintaining spinal position, push the carriage back without locking the knees, drop the heels under the bar, toe raise and then return home.

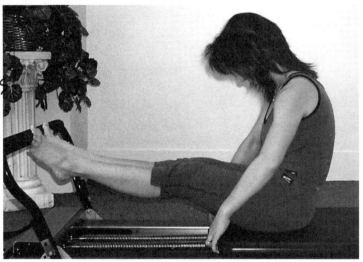

Stomach Massage Round Movement

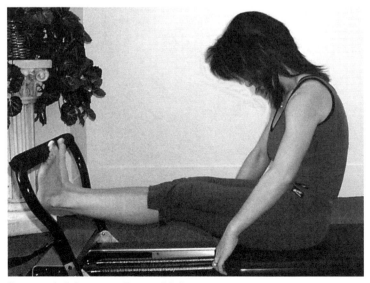

Stomach Massage Round Movement

47

STOMACH MASSAGE
Flat Back

Category: Core stability, lower body flexibility and strengthening.

Benefits: Flexibility and strengthening of the lower body, breath with movement, proximal stability and distal mobility.

Breathing: Inhale as you move the carriage back and exhale as you return home.

Prerequisites: The ability to sit in staff pose and maintain shoulder-hip alignment with a straight back.

Repetitions: 5 to 8

Springs: 1 to 2

Cues:
- Keep the knees over the second toes.
- Zip the inner thighs together as you press back.
- Keep shoulders directly over the hips throughout the movement.
- Stay on the ischial tuberosities throughout the exercise.
- Reach through the crown of your head.
- Keep your shoulders down and open to the front.

Set Up: Sit on the carriage with the balls of the feet on the footbar in "Pilates V." Sit as close to the foot-bar as you can keeping a straight spine and your shoulders over your hips. Place hands either behind you on the shoulder rests or on the carriage. Elbows stay straight, but not locked throughout the movement.

SITZ BONES

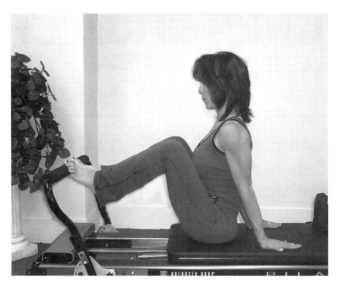
Stomach Masssage Set Up

Movement: While maintaining spinal position, push the carriage back without locking the knees, drop the heels under the bar, toe raise and then return home.

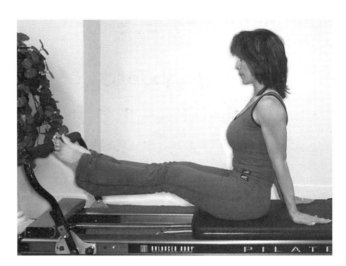
Stomach Massage Movement

Variations: Break up the motions of pushing back and calf raising into small segments for beginners. For advanced participants, have them sit in straight spine with hands off the carriage and arms in a "V" in front of their shoulders.

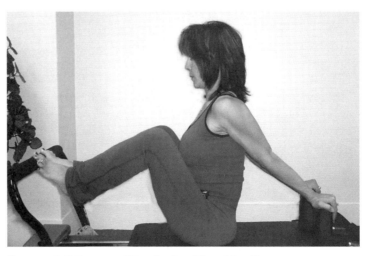
Stomach Massage Hands On Shoulder Rests

49

KNEE STRETCH SERIES
Round Back

Category: Core strengthening, lower body strengthening.

Benefits: Core and lower body strengthening, spinal flexion, breath with movement, proximal stability and distal mobility.

Breathing: Inhale as you move the carriage back and exhale as you return home.

Variations: To increase the difficulty, do the above but begin with the knees raised slightly off of the carriage.

Prerequisites: To be able to perform Cat on the mat and round the back while on all fours.

Repetitions: 8 to 10

Springs: 2 to 3 1 R + 1 B

JUST MOVE KNEES
- INHALE & HINGE c HIP
- EXHALE & SIT BUTT ↓

Cues:
- Initiate the movement at the hip joint.
- Maintain heel to knee alignment throughout the exercise.
- Keep the movement small emphasizing maintenance of round back.
- Keep your shoulders down and your back wide.

*IF shds INto EARs LOWER FtBAR
* KNEES MOVE ON ROLLERSKATES
* w/ St BACK WILL FEEL MORE ABS

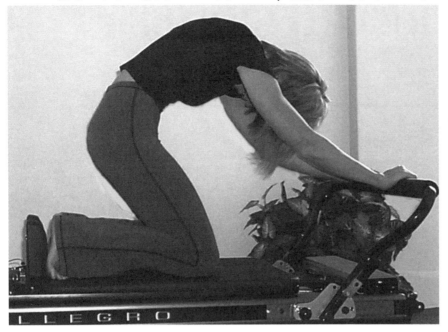

Set Up: Kneel on the carriage with your knees hip width apart, your feet against the shoulder rests and your hands shoulder width apart on the footbar. Sit back bringing your ischial tuberosities toward your heels and round your spine into flexion.

Knee Stretch Round Back Set Up

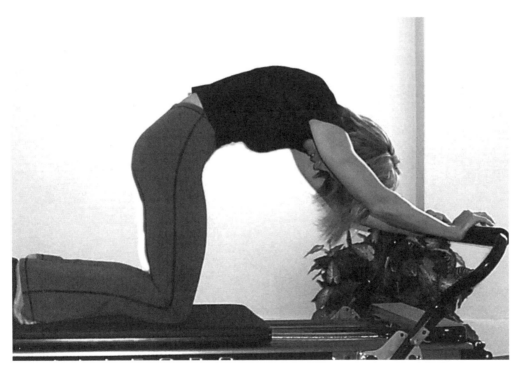

Knee Stretch Round Back Movement

Movement: While keeping your spine in flexion and your elbows extended, push the carriage back with your feet and knees. Try to bring your knees behind your hips without losing the round back position and then return the carriage using your deep abdominals.

KNEE STRETCH SERIES
Flat Back

Category: Core strengthening, lower body strengthening.

Benefits: Lower body strengthening, core stability, breath with movement, proximal stability and distal mobility.

Breathing: Inhale as you move the carriage back and exhale as you return home.

Variations: To decrease the difficulty, put the footbar down and place your hands on the sandy surface of the spring cover and perform the exercise with a neutral spine in the all fours position.

Prerequisites: The ability to hold neutral spine in all 4's position on the mat.

Repetitions: 8 to 10

Springs: 2 to 3

Cues:
- Initiate the movement at the hip joint.
- Maintain heel to knee alignment throughout the exercise.
- Keep the movement small initially emphasizing maintenance of neutral spine.
- Do not compress your lumbar spine.
- Keep your shoulders down and back.

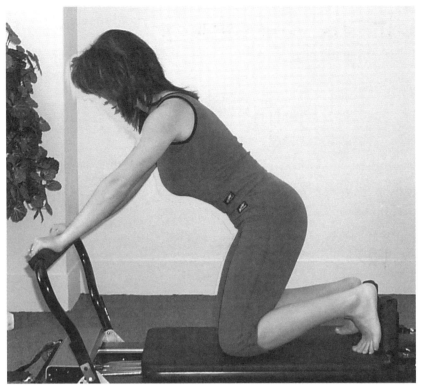

Knee Stretch Straight Set Up

Set Up: Kneel on the carriage with your knees directly under your hips, your feet against the shoulder rests and your hands shoulder width apart on the footbar. Sit back bringing your ischial tuberosities toward your heels pointing your tail bone between your legs. Maintain a neutral spine.

Movement: While keeping your spine in neutral and your elbows extended, push the carriage back with your feet and knees. Try to bring your knees directly beneath your hips without losing neutral alignment. Then return the carriage with a neutral spine.

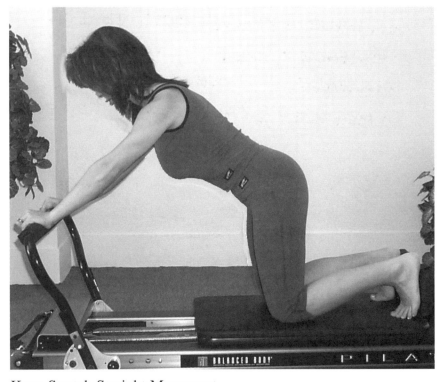

Knee Stretch Straight Movement

53

SALUTE SIT ON ~~CARRL~~ BOX

Category: Core stability, upper body strengthening.

Benefits: Stengthening of the upper body, powerhouse stability.

Breathing: Inhale as you reach your arms forward. Exhale as you return.

Variations: Reverse the breathing to add variety. Beginners can sit with their legs crossed.

Prerequisites: Rowing series on the mat. The ability to sit and maintain a straight back with spinal neutral while moving extremities.

Repetitions: 5 to 8

Springs: 1 to 2 1R or 1B

- DRAW IN RIBCAGE
- INHALE PUSH OUT
- EXHALE COME IN

VARIATION: OFFERING

START BICEP CURL POSITION (PALMS UP)
- INHALE - PRESS OUT TO FORWARD
- EXHALE - OPEN TO ALd
- INHALE - CLOSE TO CtR
- EXHALE - DRAW ARMS TO STARTING

Cues:

- Stay on the ischial tuberosities as you press the hands forward.
- Keep your back straight as you press in and out.
- Do not allow your shoulders to elevate when pressing out.
- Move only at the elbow, keep your spine neutral and stable.

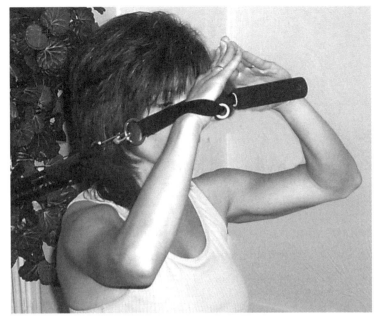

Set Up: Sit on the carriage facing the footbar with your buttocks against the shoulder rests. Extend your legs in front of you and place the backs of your hands against your forehead while holding onto the handles. Sit in straight back with your shoulders and hips aligned.

Salute Set Up

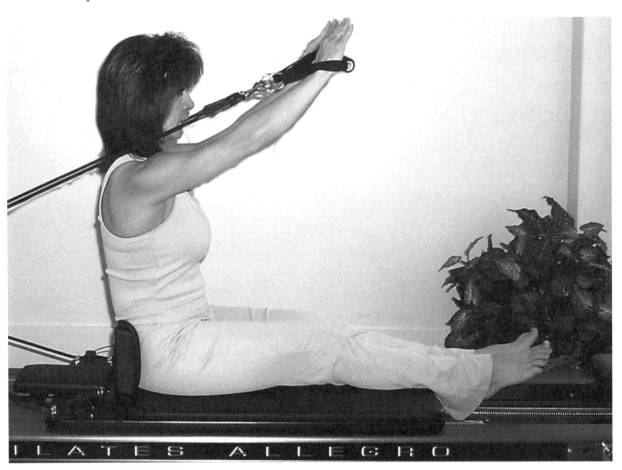

Salute Movement

Movement: Extend your elbows, while keeping spinal neutral and your shoulders down your back. Return to the starting position with control.

ROWING FRONT SERIES
Tree Hug

Category: Upper body strengthening, core stability.

Benefits: Strengthening of the upper body, flexibility of the lower body, core and shoulder stability, breath with movement, proximal stability and distal mobility.

Breathing: Inhale as you draw your fingers together and exhale as you open for the first 3 repetitions. Then reverse the breath to exhale coming together for the second 3 repetitions.

Variations: Beginners may do this exercise in a cross legged position.

Prerequisites: The ability to maintain shoulder-hip alignment in a seated position while moving the upper body.

Repetitions: 5 to 8

Springs: 1 to 2   1 B OR 1 R (IF STRONG)

- INHALE CLOSE TOGETHER
- EXHALE OPEN
  (HUG A TREE)

Cues:
- Keep your ischial tuberosities firmly on the carriage.
- Press into the carriage with your knees in the cross legged position.
- Keep the back straight, spine stable, and the shoulders over the hips.
- Reach long through the crown of your head.
- Stay heavy in your armpit and slightly raise your elbows.
- Keep your shoulders down and open to the front.

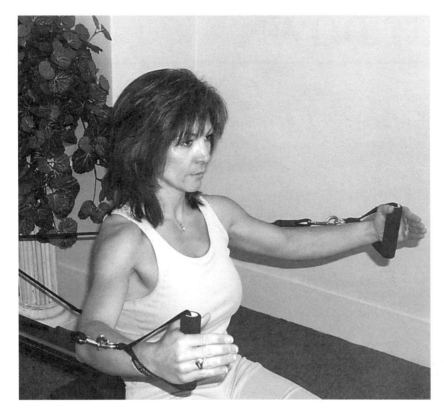

Set Up: Long sit on the carriage facing the footbar, with your back against the shoulder rests. Sit tall with a straight back and hold the small loops or handles in your hands. Slightly bend your elbows and abduct the arms to shoulder height. Raise the elbows slightly higher than the hands to keep the back wide and the scapula down.

Tree Hug Set Up

Movement: Maintain a straight back as you close your hands like you are hugging a tree. Return the arms to the open position without allowing the elbows to extend behind the shoulders.

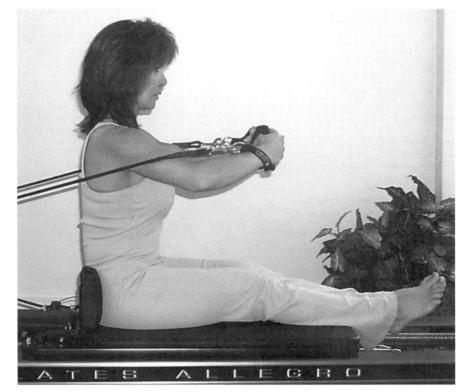

Tree Hug Movement

CHEST OUT DOWN

Category: Upper body strengthening, core stability.

Benefits: Scapular stabilization, flexibility and strengthening of the upper body, awareness of spinal neutral in a seated position, breath with movement, proximal stability and distal mobility.

Breathing: Inhale as arms extend and exhale as you return home.

Variations: As you get more advanced, sit with your legs extended in a long sitting position.

Prerequisites: The ability to long sit (staff pose).

Repetitions: 5 to 8

Springs: 1 to 2   I R OR IB

· INHALE - ARMS OUT

EXHALE PRESS ↓

    CIRCLE TO ↑

· DO TREE HUGGER AFTER

Cues:
- Start with your hips and shoulders aligned.
- Keep your hands open and your shoulders relaxed.
- Keep your back straight and reach out through the crown of your head.
- Do not let your arms go behind your shoulders when circling.
- Protract the shoulders throughout the movement.

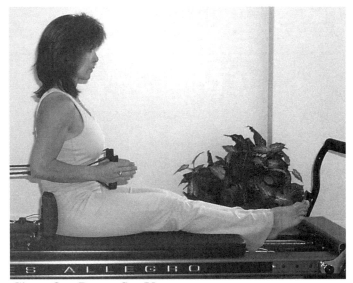

Chest Out Down Set Up

Set Up: Long sit with your back against the shoulder rests. Place your hands in the small loops with your palms against your ribcage. Keep your back straight and your elbows facing to the back.

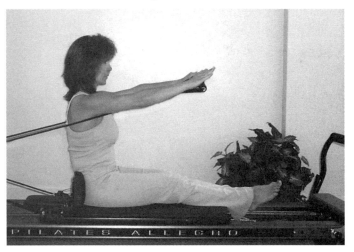

Chest Out Down Movement

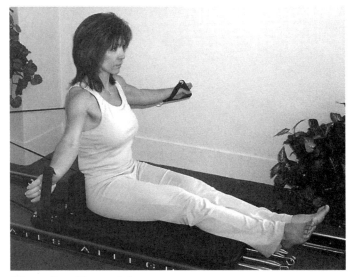

Chest Out Down Movement

Movement: Extend your arms forward at the level of your shoulders. Lower your hands and then circle the shoulders upwards returning to the starting position.

ROWING BACK

Category: Upper body strengthening, core stability.

Benefits: Scapular stabilization, strengthening of the upper body and core, spinal flexion.

Breathing: Exhale as you round back and inhale as you return.

Variations: For advanced participants, do bicep curls while in the rounded back position. To decrease the difficulty place your knuckles together and hold in front of your sternum. Maintain this position as you roll back and up.

Prerequisites: Roll up on the mat.

Repetitions: 5 to 8

Springs: 1 to 2   1 R OR 1 B

FOCUS ON C CURVE

RETURN 3/4 WAY AS LONG AS BACK IS ROUNDED

Cues:
- Keep your elbows in line with your shoulders ✔ throughout entire exercise.
- Use the abdominals to round the spine down and up.
- Keep your scapulae down your back.

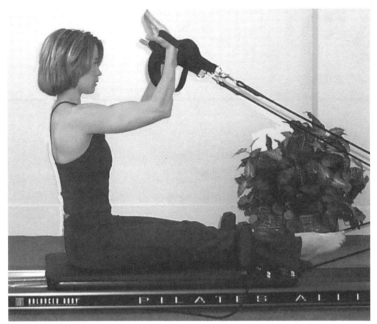
Roll Back Set up

Set Up: Sit on the carriage facing the head rest with legs between shoulder rests in a long sit. Place the lower body in "Pilates V". Hands are in the small loops with both arms bent at a 90 degree angle in front of the chest. The elbows are in line with the shoulders and the palms are facing the body.

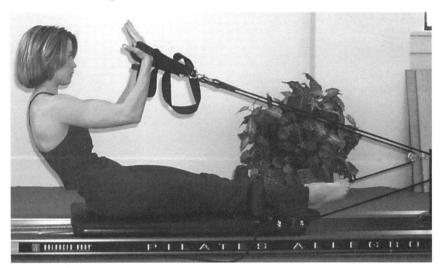
Roll Back Movement

Movement: While keeping the arms up, round the back, scoop the abdominals and roll back. Keep arms up and roll slowly back to the beginning position.

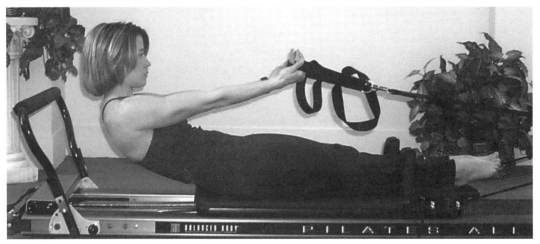
Roll Back with Bicep Curl

KNEELING ARM SIDE
Rotation

Category: Core stability, upper body strengthening and flexibility.

Benefits: Strengthening of the rotator cuff and powerhouse, proximal stability and distal mobility.

Breathing: Inhale as you pull the rope and exhale as you release it.

Variations: For beginners, place feet together forming a triangle to increase the base of support. For the more advanced, move away from the shoulder rests.

Prerequisites: Awareness of neutral in a kneeling position.

Repetitions: 5 to 8

Springs: 1 to 2   *1R OR 1B OR 1Y*

• INHALE PULL ACROSS
• EXHALE - RELEASE

Cues:
- Do not allow your back to arch during the movement.
- Keep your shoulders open and down as you move the arm.
- Keep your tailbone between your legs.
- Align your heels directly behind your knees.

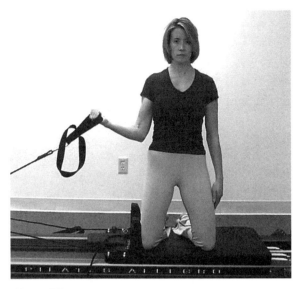 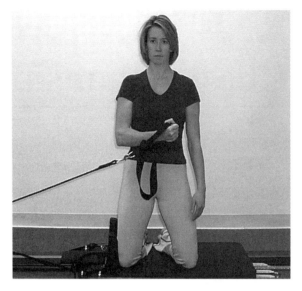

Set Up: INTERNAL ROTATION—Kneel on the carriage with the side of your right leg against the shoulder rests. Place your knees hip width apart. Grasp one handle with the right hand. Place your shoulders directly in line with your hips, and keep the front of your shoulder open to the wall in front of you.

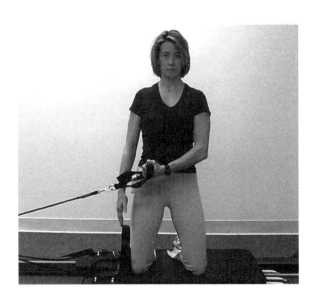 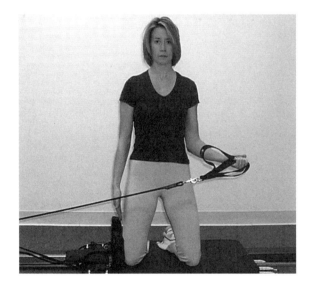

Set Up: EXTERNAL ROTATION—Kneel on the carriage with the side of your right leg against the shoulder rests and your knees hip width apart. Grasp the handle with the left hand with the palm facing to the ceiling. Place your shoulders directly in line with your hips, and keep the front of your shoulder open to the wall in front of you.

Movement: Keep your elbow next to your ribs and your shoulders down and relaxed. Pull the rope toward your abdomen (internal) or away from you (external).

63

KNEELING ARM SERIES
Chest Expansion

Category: Upper body strengthening, core stability.

Benefits: Strengthening and flexibility of the upper body, awareness of spinal neutral while in a kneeling position, breath with movement, proximal stability and distal mobility.

Breathing: Inhale as you move the carriage back and exhale as you return home.

Variations: Allow beginners to sit on their heels and have more advanced participants kneel in the center of the carriage with their feet hooked over the edge of the carriage.

Prerequisites: The ability to hold spinal and pelvic neutral while in a kneeling position.

Repetitions: 5 to 8

Springs: 1 to 2   1R OR 1B

· INHALE to PULL BACK

TO MODIFY - SIT ON BOX

Cues:
- Keep your knees directly under hips, and shoulders in line with your hips.
- Keep your chest open, neutral spine and your upper back wide.
- Maintain shoulder to hip alignment throughout the exercise.
- Reach through the crown of your head.
- Draw your shoulders down.

Set Up: Kneel on the carriage with your knees against the shoulder rests. Feet flexed and heels in line with the sitz bones. Hold onto either the small loops or the rope above the metal clips with your arms at your sides and palms facing toward your body.

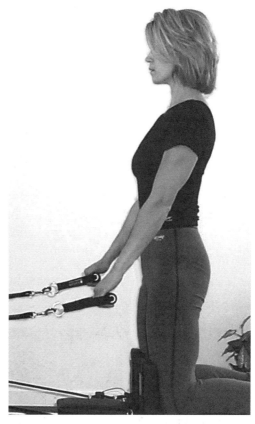

Chest Expansion Set Up

Movement: Keeping your elbows straight, pull the straps to your sides by extending your shoulders. Hold this position while you turn your head left, center, and right. Return to the set up position with control.

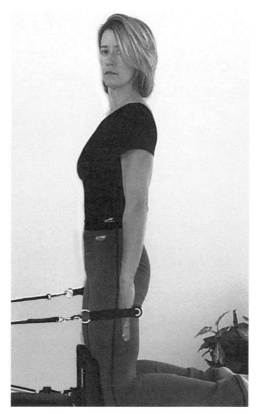

Chest Expansion Movement

SHORT BOX SERIES
Round Back

Category: Core strengthening.

Benefits: Powerhouse strengthening, lumbar flexibility.

Breathing: Exhale as you round your spine and draw your navel in. Inhale as you return to the starting position.

Variations: To decrease the difficulty, leave arms at your sides. To increase the difficulty, hold a dowel rod with the arms fully extended in front of your shoulders or above your head.

Prerequisites: Spine stretch and roll up on mat. Rowing back roll back on the reformer.

Repetitions: 8 to 10

Springs: 4 (ALL SPRINGS)

HOLD POLE W/ ARMS WIDE

• EXHALE - RD BACK

*• DO PELVIC TUCKS FIRST

Cues:
- Draw your navel to your spine.
- Avoid internal or external rotation of the hips during movement.
- Widen the back and soften the neck.
- Keep a space between your chin and chest.

Set Up: Place the box horizontally on carriage against the shoulder rests. Attach the footstrap and hook all springs. Sit on the box with one hand width behind you and place your feet under the strap. Extend your arms in front of you at shoulder height and begin in neutral spine.

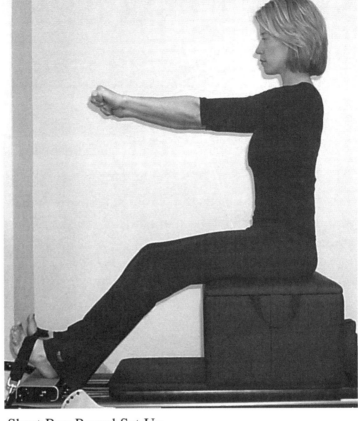

Short Box Round Set Up

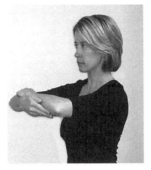

Arm Variation

Movement: Round your spine and roll back as if you were lying your vertebrae to the box one at a time. Continue back until you are unable to hold alignment and then, return to the starting position.

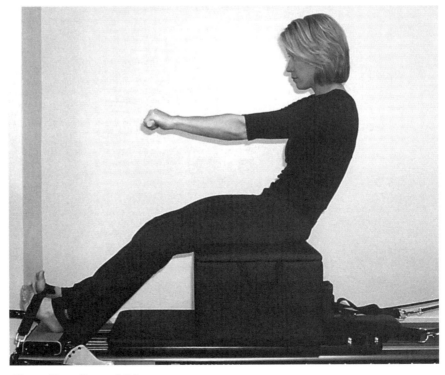

Short Box Round Movement

SHORT BOX SERIES
Tilt

Category: Core stability and strengthening.

Benefits: Powerhouse stability, strengthening of quadratus lumborum, spinal mobility.

Breathing: Exhale as you sidebend and inhale as you return to the starting position.

Variations: To increase the difficulty, use a weighted rod. To decrease the difficulty, place your hands behind your head or put your arms in front of you "genie" style.

Prerequisites: Mermaid on the mat or the reformer. Short box round and straight on the reformer.

Repetitions: 8 to 10

Springs: 4

Cues:

- Draw your navel to your spine.
- Avoid internal or external rotation of the hips during movement.
- Widen the back and soften the neck.
- Keep the pelvis firmly planted on the box and the ribcage in line with the front wall.
- Keep lifting and lengthening the spine throughout the movement.

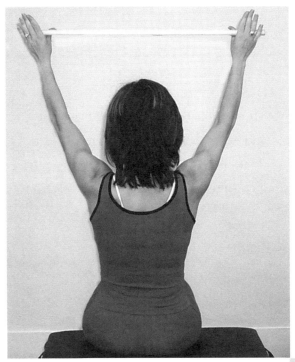

Short Box Tilt Set Up

Set Up: Place box horizontally on carriage against the shoulder rests. Attach the foot-strap and hook all springs. Sit on the box with one hand width behind you and place your feet under the strap. Hold a dowel rod over head with the arms fully extended.

Movement: Sidebend to one side keeping the ischial tuberosities on the box and creating a "C" curve of the spine from head to hip. Return to center reaching long in your torso, and then go to the other side. Maintain a neutral pelvis throughout the movement.

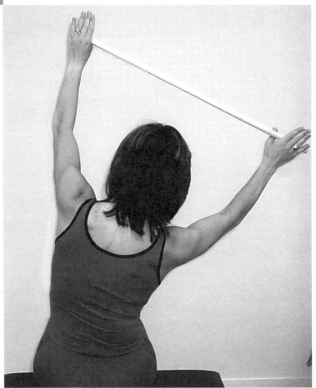

Short Box Tilt Movement

SIDE SPLIT

Category: Lower body strengthening and flexibility, core stability.

Benefits: Flexibility and strengthening of the lower body, balance and powerhouse stability.

Breathing: Inhale as you move the carriage back and exhale as you return home.

Variations: Do the same with the hips in external rotation and feet in line with the patella. To increase the difficulty, bend over to touch the side rail while the carriage is open. Return to the standing position before bringing the carriage home. You may also hold a gondola pole if needed for balance.

Prerequisites: The ability to hold neutral in a standing position.

Repetitions: 8 to 10

Springs: 1 to 2

Cues:

- Avoid hyperextension of the knees.
- Reach tall through the crown of your head.
- Feel a wrapping sensation in the buttocks as you draw your legs together.
- Widen the back and soften the neck.

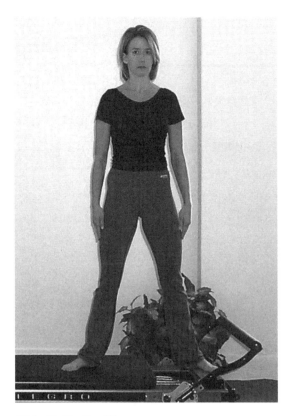

Side Split Set Up

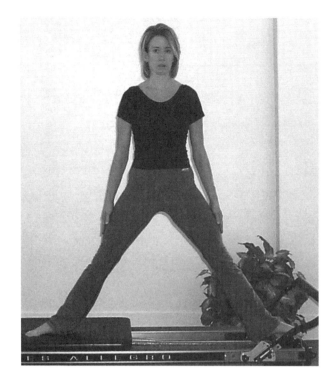

Side Split Movement

Set Up: Stand on the carriage with one foot on the sandy surface of the footplate and the other against the shoulder rest. Align your second toe with your patella with your feet in a forward position. Keep your tail bone pointing down and the pelvis and spine in neutral. Hold your arms out to the sides at shoulder height to assist with balance.

Movement: Push the carriage back while gently internally rotating the femurs. Return the carriage with control as you gently externally rotate the hips and raise the pelvic floor.

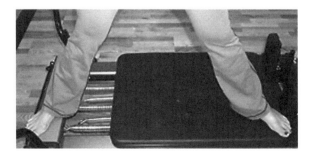

Side Split Hips in External Rotation

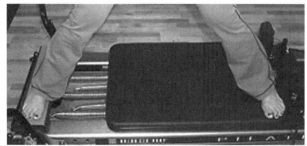

Side Split Neutral

EVE'S LUNGE

Category: Lower body flexibility and strengthening, core stability.

Benefits: Flexibility and strengthening of the lower body, awareness of spinal neutral in a standing position, proximal stability and distal mobility, unilateral movement.

Breathing: Inhale as you move the carriage back and exhale as you return home.

Variations: If your reformer is not on legs, stand and place your foot on the shoulder rest. Use a gondola pole for balance as you will not be able to hold the footbar with your hands.

Prerequisites: The ability to perform a low lunge on the floor while maintaining shoulder-hip alignment and keeping your ASIS pointing forward.

Repetitions: 8 to 10

Springs: 1 to 2

> ## Cues:
> - Maintain a neutral spine and keep your pelvis in line with the wall in front of you.
> - Reach long through the top back of your head.
> - Widen the back and soften the neck.
> - Do not let your knee go past your toe on the supporting leg.
> - Keep the ASIS in the same transverse plane.

Set Up: Kneel on the carriage with one foot flat against the shoulder rest. Footbar is in the highest position. Place the other leg on the floor next to the footbar. Line up the heel of the foot on the carriage with the knee and ischial tuberosities. Align your pelvis and shoulder girdle with the wall in front of you.

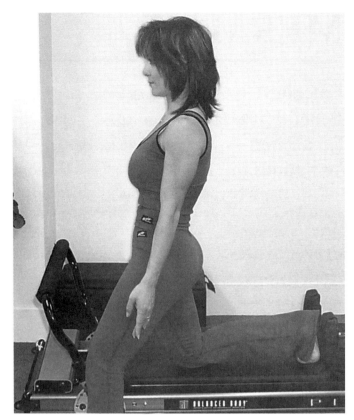

Eve's Lunge Set Up

Movement: Push the carriage back, initiating from the hips, as far as you can without losing neutral spine. Return the carriage with control.

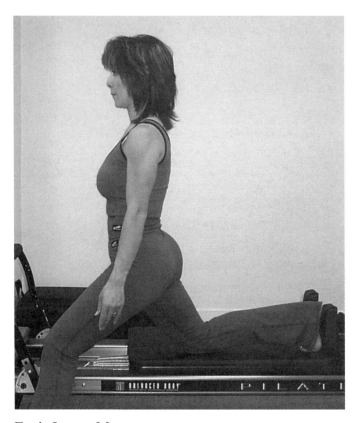

Eve's Lunge Movement

73

MERMAID

Category: Core strengthening and flexibility.

Benefits: Flexibility and strengthening of the powerhouse, breath with movement.

Breathing: Inhale as you move the carriage back and exhale as you return home.

Variations: For less difficulty sit cross legged, and as you progress begin sitting on one hip with the knees separated. As flexibility improves, bring the knees over one another into a stacked position. In this stacked position, you can also hold the carriage out and lift your hips up off of the carriage.

Prerequisites: Mermaid on the mat with the ability to hold neutral while side-bending.

Repetitions: 8 to 10

Springs: 1 to 2

Cues:
- Keep the ischial tuberosities on the carriage throughout the movement.
- Lengthen your spine and keep reaching your upper extremities toward the ceiling and side walls.
- Keep your ribcage square to the wall in front of you, avoiding spinal rotation.

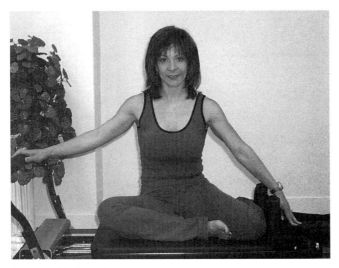

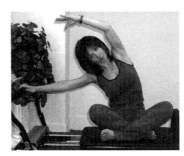

Mermaid Less Flexibility

Mermaid Set Up

Set Up: Sit on the carriage facing one side with your left shin toward the shoulder rests and your right hip toward the foot bar. Place one hand on the footbar and the other on your shin. Align your ribcage with the wall in front of you and place both ischial tuberosities on the carriage.

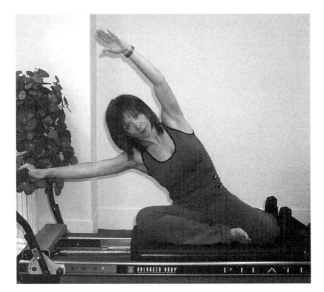

Mermaid Movement

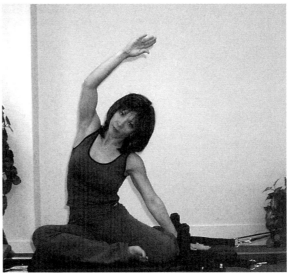

Mermaid Movement

Movement: Push the carriage back as you side bend into a "C" curve toward the footbar and bring your arm overhead. Allow the carriage to slowly return to home. When the carriage is parked side bend on the opposite side into a "C" curve toward the shoulder rests with your arm reaching overhead.

RUNNING

Category: Warm up, cool down.

Benefits: Heat builder, flexibility and strengthening of the lower body, awareness of spinal neutral, breath with movement, proximal stability and distal mobility.

Breathing: Keep the breath even with the length of the inhale equal to the length of the exhale.

Variations: Push off with bent knee leg for quadricep work and the straight knee for calf work.

Prerequisites: The ability to maintain spinal and pelvic neutral during movement.

Repetitions: 8 to 10

Springs: 3 to 4

Cues:

- Keep the knees over the second toes.
- Keep the knees pointing toward the ceiling (avoid femoral anteversion).
- Stay in neutral spine.
- Widen the back and soften the neck.
- Press evenly through both feet (avoid pronating or supinating the feet).

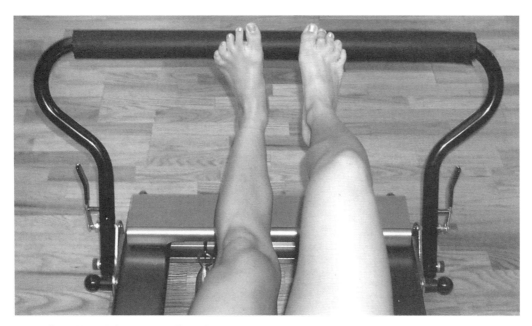

Running Foot Placement Set Up

Set Up: Lie supine on the carriage with the head rest up and the pelvis and ribcage in neutral. Place the balls of the feet on the footbar with the toes curled softly over and feet parallel.

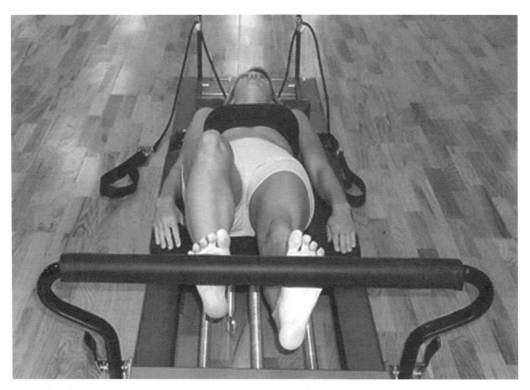

Running Movement

Movement: Push the carriage back with both legs softly extending the knees. Start by lowering one heel under the bar and then the opposite one. Alternate back and forth.

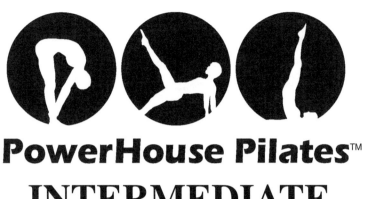

PowerHouse Pilates™
INTERMEDIATE
REFORMER EXERCISES

This section will help you progress your existing Pilates clientele using intermediate exercises and additional accessories. Many of the intermediate exercises listed are an extension of the beginning exercises. Once you have learned the components in the beginning exercises it will become very easy to add the intermediate exercises into your repertoire for group or private Pilates reformer training.

Once you have mastered Sections 1 & 2 you will have many exercises and variations to keep your Pilates reformer program going strong for years. Remember our clients aren't getting bored, we are! Use the many variations available with each exercise to keep adding interest and variety to your Pilates reformer program. Carefully progress your clients into the intermediate exercises by adding a new exercise each session.

"Man should bear in mind and ponder over the Greek—not too much, not too little."

Joseph Pilates

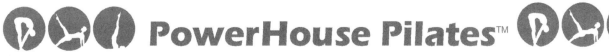 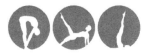

UPSTRETCH

Category: Core stability and strengthening, upper and lower body strengthening.

Benefits: Flexibility and strengthening of the upper and lower body, strengthening and stability of the Powerhouse, breath with movement.

Breathing: Inhale as you move the carriage back and exhale as you return home.

Variations: For emphasis on posture do this exercise with a straight back, flattening the thoracic spine. For abdominal emphasis, use a slightly rounded back. Try reversing the progression of movements for challenge and interest. For beginners, break the movement into pieces.

Prerequisites: Long stretch, arabesque, and elephant on the reformer. Plank and leg pull front on the mat.

Repetitions: 8 to 10

Springs: 2 to 3

Cues:
- Keep the ischial tuberosities toward the ceiling.
- Return carriage softly to full park position before beginning again.
- Maintain the neck as a natural extension of the spine.
- Widen the back and keep the serratus anterior engaged.

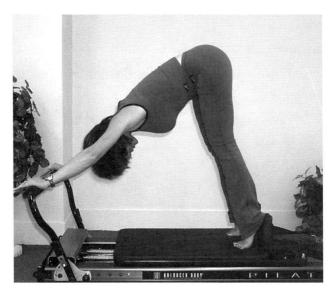

Upstretch Set Up

Set Up: Place balls of the feet on the carriage with the heels against the shoulder rests and hands shoulder width apart on the footbar. Keep the thumbs with the fingers, press the chest toward the thighs and the ischial tuberosities toward the ceiling.

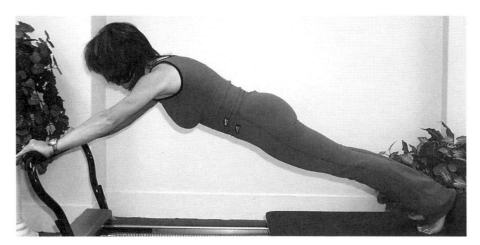

Upstretch Movement

Movement: Push the carriage back as you extend the hips into a plank position. Come forward over the footbar while maintaining the plank as you would in long stretch. Keep your hands in line with your shoulders. Bring the carriage to a parked position by returning to the starting position.

81

ARABESQUE

Category: Core stability and strengthening, upper and lower body strengthening and flexibility.

Benefits: Powerhouse stability and strengthening, flexibility of the thoracic spine and lower extremities, breath with movement.

Breathing: Inhale as you push the carriage backward and exhale as you return.

Variations: Reverse the breathing to add variation. To create length and flexibility in the thoracic spine do this exercise with a straight back, to emphasize abdominal work do this exercise with a slightly rounded spine. If weight shifts to one side reduce the spring tension.

Prerequisites: Elephant on the reformer and push up on the mat.

Repetitions: 3 to 5

Springs: 1 to 2

Cues:

- Focus on drawing your leg back and controlling the movement utilizing the abdominals.
- Keep the ischial tuberosities to the ceiling.
- Shoulder blades should be flat against the back.
- Keep your range of motion small to control the movement.
- Keep your ASIS pointing forward during the movement.
- Equalize weight between the upper extremities.

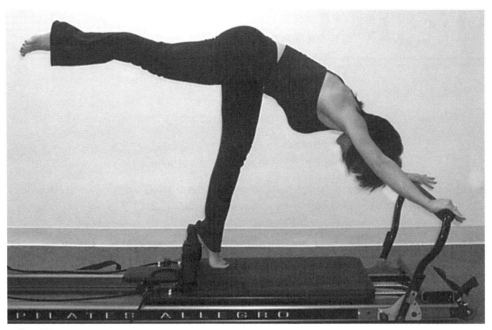

Arabesque Set Up

Set Up: Place the balls of the feet on the carriage with the heels against the shoulder rest and hands shoulder width apart on the footbar. Keep the thumbs with the fingers. Press the chest toward the thighs and the ischial tuberosities toward the ceiling. Keep your ears between your elbows, and lengthen your spine to a flat back. Extend one leg behind you, pointing your toe softly.

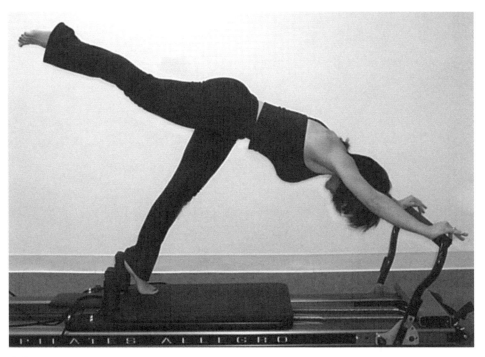

Arabesque Movement

Movement: Push the carriage back with the foot on the carriage keeping the body in an upside-down "V". Hinge at the hips as far as you can maintaining spinal alignment. Keeping the lifted leg extended behind you. Return to the starting position in a controlled movement.

SEMICIRCLE

Category: Core stability and lower body flexibility.

Benefits: Flexibility and strengthening of the lower body and the Powerhouse, awareness of spinal neutral, breath with movement.

Breathing: Inhale as you move the carriage back and exhale as you return home.

Variations: Do this version 4 times and then reverse the circle for 4 repetitions. For beginners, widen the feet to hip width apart still keeping the knee and second toe aligned. Hips will be slightly externally rotated.

Prerequisites: Pelvic lift and Eve's lunge on the reformer. Articulating bridge and shoulder bridge on the mat.

Repetitions: 8 to 10

Springs: 2 to 4

Cues:
- Keep the knees over the second toe and the heels pressed tightly together.
- Zip the inner thighs together as you press back.
- Feel a wrapping sensation in the buttocks.
- Widen the back and soften the neck.
- Keep the ribcage in neutral (avoid "boinking" the 10th rib).
- Keep your shoulders down and wide.

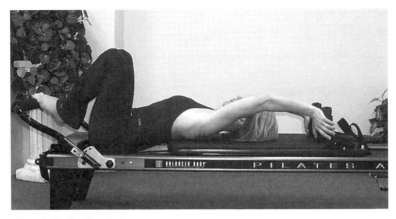

Semicircle Set Up

Set Up: For this exercise the footbar will need to be in the lowest position. Lie supine on the carriage with the balls of the feet on the footbar in "Pilates V". Slide your upper body down the carriage as you press back so that your elbows are fully extended with your hands against the shoulder rests. Bend your knees and drop your buttocks into the springs with slight lumbar extension.

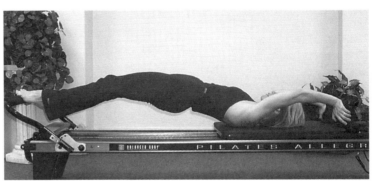

Semicircle Movement

Movement: Push the carriage back without locking the knees, keep the carriage still as you bridge the spine from the carriage. Return the carriage home with the buttocks lifted and send the knees out over the footbar for a hip flexor stretch while maintaining the "Pilates V". Keep the carriage still as you return to the starting position.

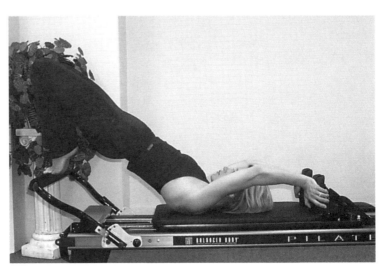

Semicircle Movement

85

LONG SPINE

Category: Core strengthening.

Benefits: Powerhouse strengthening, flexibility of the spine and lower body, breath with movement.

Breathing: Exhale as you extend your legs to the ceiling, and inhale as you roll back onto the carriage.

Variations: For variety, open the legs to shoulder width as you would for a rollover on the mat or place your feet parallel instead of "Pilates V". You can also reverse your breathing. For more stretch, place your feet in the small loops.

Prerequisites: Rollover, articulating bridge, and double leg stretch on mat. Short spine and leg circles on the reformer.

Repetitions: 8 to 10

Springs: 2 to 4

Cues:

- Zip and wrap the lower extremities together as you lower the legs to the set up position.
- Do not roll onto your neck.
- Widen the back and soften the neck.
- Keep space between your ribcage and pelvis.
- Don't miss the lower back when articulating the spine back onto the carriage.

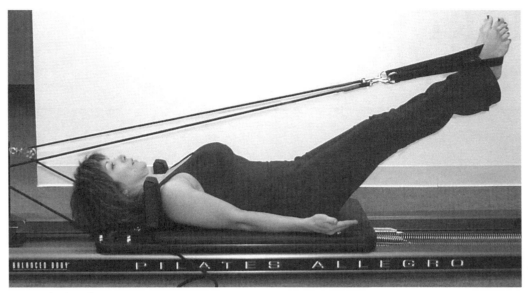

Long Spine Set Up

Set Up: Lie supine on the carriage with the head rest down, your feet in the large loops, and your lower extremities extended, wrapped and zipped into "Pilates V". Pelvis and ribcage should be in neutral and the carriage will be in the pushed back position.

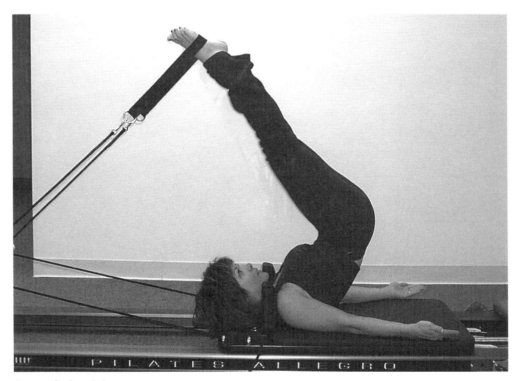

Long Spine Movement

Movement: Begin by peeling your spine off of the carriage while keeping your feet extended toward the ceiling in "Pilates V". When you reach your shoulder blades, slowly curl your spine back onto the carriage one vertebrae at a time. After the sacrum touches the carriage, lower the legs to the starting position and the pelvis back to neutral.

SHORT BOX SERIES
Straight Back

Category: Core stability.

Benefits: Powerhouse stability.

Breathing: Exhale as you hinge backward, inhale in the extended position, then exhale as you return to the starting position.

Variations: To decrease the difficulty, leave arms at your sides. To increase the difficulty, hold a dowel rod with the arms fully extended above your head or slightly in front of your torso. To help the participant visualize place the dowel rod along their spine as they hinge backward.

Prerequisites: Rowing back series, chest out down, and short box round on the reformer.

Repetitions: 8 to 10

Springs: 4

Cues:
- Draw your navel to your spine.
- Avoid internal or external rotation of the hips during movement.
- Widen the back and soften the neck.
- Reach out through the crown of your head.
- Avoid compressing your low back.

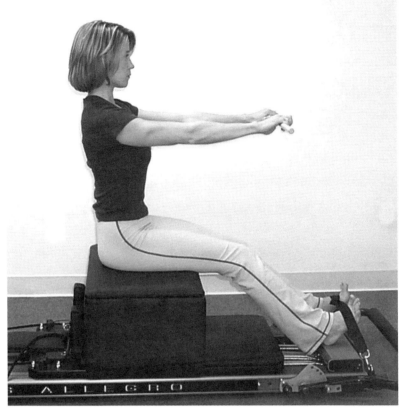

Set Up: Place box horizontally on carriage against the shoulder rests. Attach the footstrap and hook all springs. Sit on the box with one hand width behind you and place your feet under the strap. Extend your arms in front of you at shoulder height and begin in neutral spine.

Short Box Straight Set Up

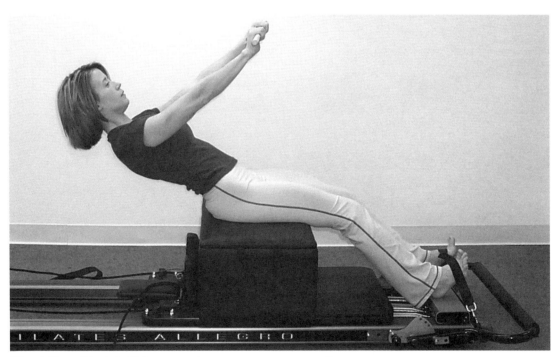

Short Box Straight Movement

Movement: Hinge backward from the hip joint with a neutral spine. Go as far as you can while maintaining the neutral spine and then return to the starting position.

SHORT BOX SERIES
Tilt / Twist

Category: Core strengthening.

Benefits: Powerhouse strengthening and flexibility, especially of the obliques.

Breathing: Exhale as you sidebend and twist; inhale as you return to the starting position.

Variations: To increase the difficulty, use a weighted rod and extend the rod and point behind you. To decrease the difficulty, place your hands behind your head or hold arms "genie" style.

Prerequisites: Saw on the mat. Short box series and stomach massage twist on the reformer.

Repetitions: 8 to 10

Springs: 4

Cues:
- Draw your navel to your spine.
- Avoid internal or external rotation of the hips during movement.
- Widen the back and soften the neck.
- Keep the pelvis firmly planted on the box.

Set Up: Place box horizontally on carriage against the shoulder rests. Attach footstrap and hook all springs. Sit on the box with one hand width behind you and place your feet under the strap. Hold a dowel rod over head with the arms fully extended and hands slightly in front of your shoulders.

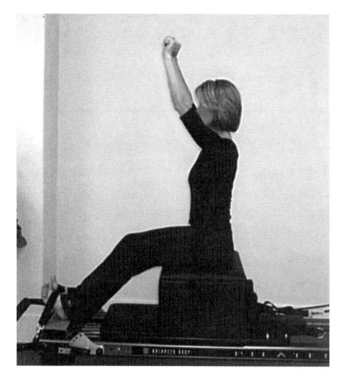

Short Box Tilt Twist Set Up

M o v e m e n t : Simultaneously sidebend and twist to one side keeping the ischial tuberosities on the box. When you have gone back as far as you can without losing neutral pelvis, return to the starting position. Continue to the other side.

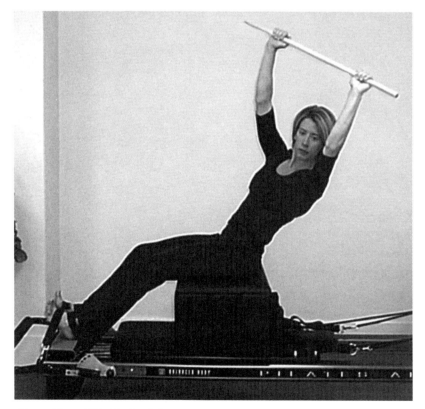

Short Box Tilt Twist Movement

LONG BOX SERIES
T-Press

Category: Upper body strengthening.

Benefits: Strengthening of the mid and upper back and upper extremities, lengthening of the cervical and lumbar spine, awareness of spinal neutral in the prone position, breath with movement, proximal stability and distal mobility.

Breathing: Inhale as you pull the straps and exhale as you return to the starting position.

Variations: Try hands in the loops or use handles if the wrists are unstable or grip is weak.

Prerequisites: Swimming or flight on the mat.

Repetitions: 8 to 10

Springs: 1 to 2

Cues:
- Keep the pubic bone on the box and do not hyperextend the lumbar spine.
- Reach long through the crown of your head to avoid cervical hyperextension.
- Widen the back and soften the neck.
- Do not allow the hands to raise higher than 90^0 of shoulder abduction.

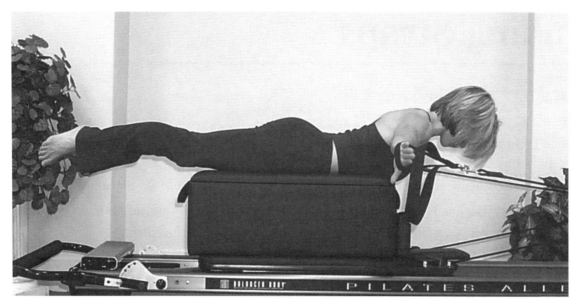

Long Box T-Press Set Up

Set Up: Place the box in the long position with one end against the shoulder rests. Lie on the box with your manubrium extending beyond the front end of the box and your hands in the small loops. Extend your arms directly out to the sides just below shoulder height with the hands in pronation.

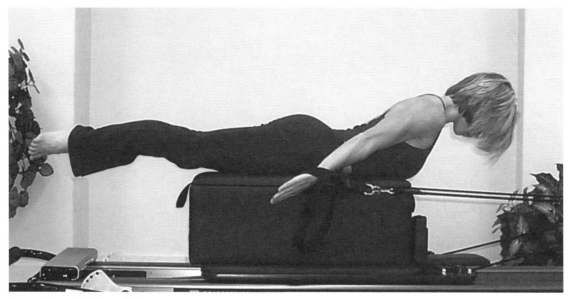

Long Box T-Press Movement

Movement: Pull the straps into your sides with the elbows extended, and then return to the starting position.

LONG BOX SERIES
Pulling Straps

Category: Upper body strengthening.

Benefits: Strengthening of the mid and upper back and upper extremities, lengthening of the cervical and lumbar spine, awareness of spinal neutral in the prone position, breath with movement, proximal stability and distal mobility.

Breathing: Inhale as you pull the straps and exhale as you return to the starting position.

Variations: Try hands in the loops or use handles if the wrists are unstable or grip is weak. As you get stronger, drop the head and upper body as you return the carriage.

Prerequisites: Flight and double leg kick on mat.

Repetitions: 8 to 10

Springs: 1 to 2

Cues:
- Keep the pubic bone on the box and do not hyperextend the lumbar spine.
- Reach long through the crown of your head to avoid cervical hyperextension.
- Widen the back and soften the neck.
- Imagine paddling a canoe without oars.

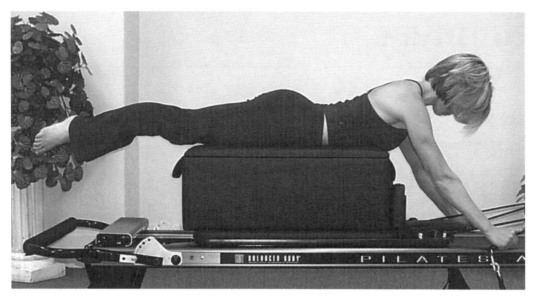

Long Box Pull Straps Set Up

Set Up: Place the box in the long position with one end against the shoulder rests. Lie on long box with your manubrium extending beyond the front end of the box and your hands holding the straps just above the loop clip. Drop your upper extremities toward the floor on the outside of the side rails while keeping the straps taut. Keep the spine in neutral, and the legs and buttocks active.

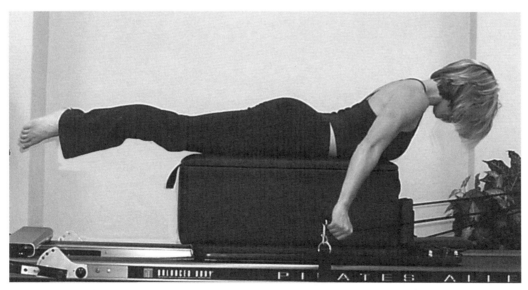

Long Box Pull Straps Movement

Movement: Pull the straps back with the elbows extended until your arms reach your sides, and then return to the starting position.

LONG BOX SERIES
Swimming

Category: Core stability and strengthening. Upper and lower body strengthening and stability.

Benefits: Strengthening of the powerhouse, balance, spinal flexibility and awareness of neutral in a prone position.

Breathing: Inhale for a count a four and exhale for four.

Variations: Have beginners break up the movement, using only their arms or their legs.

Prerequisites: Swimming on the mat.

Repetitions: 8 to 10

Springs: All

Cues:
- Keep the pubic bone on the box.
- Do not hyperextend the lumbar spine.
- Reach through the crown of your head.
- Widen the back and keep the shoulders down.
- Do not rock your torso back and forth.

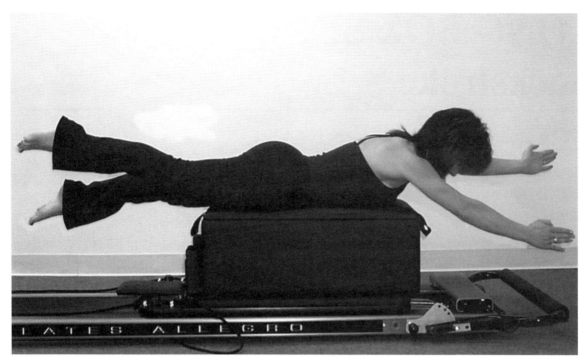

Long Box Series Swimming

Set Up: Place the box in the long position with the short end against the shoulder rests. Lie on the box with your manubrium extending beyond the front end of the box. Press your pubic bone into the box. Reach the crown of your head for the wall in front of you and reach your feet for the wall behind you.

Movement: While holding your torso still, raise your opposite arm and leg. Keep pressing your pubic bone into the box, and lengthen the arms and legs in opposition to the torso. Keep alternating back and forth.

LONG BOX SERIES
Backstroke

Category: Upper body strengthening and core stability.

Benefits: Strengthening of the abdominals and upper extremities, awareness of spinal neutral in the supine position, breath with movement, proximal stability and distal mobility.

Breathing: Inhale as you pull the straps and exhale as you return to the starting position.

Variations: For beginners, circle just the arms while stabilizing your torso on the box or shorten the levers by bending at the elbows and knees. For more advanced participants, draw your legs in first and then draw in your arms. To add variety reverse the circle.

Prerequisites: Double leg stretch on mat. Hundred position, leg circles and arm circles on the reformer.

Repetitions: 8 to 10

Springs: 1 to 2

Cues:
- Keep your head and shoulders lifted as you perform the movement.
- Keep the powerhouse stabilized as you perform the movement.
- Do not circle your arms behind your shoulders.
- Reach your arms and legs for the walls to lengthen as you circle.

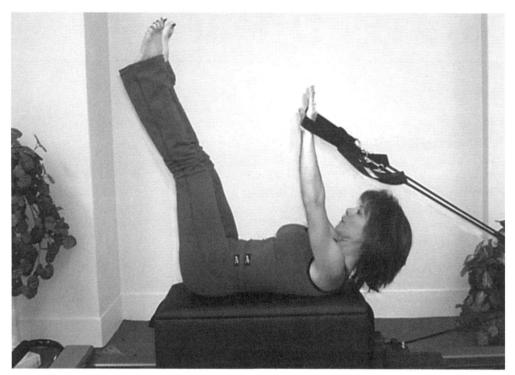

Back Stroke Set Up

Set Up: Place the box in the long position with one end against the shoulder rests. Lie supine on the box with your hands in the handles. Place your pelvis and ribcage in neutral. Extend your arms and legs toward the ceiling keeping them directly above the hip and shoulder joints. Keeping your tailbone on the box, roll up into the hundred position.

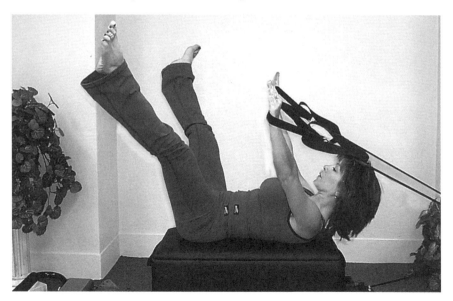

Back Stroke Movement

Movement: While maintaining proximal stability, open your arms and legs and circle them at the same time as if you were performing a backstroke while swimming. Return your arms and legs to the beginning position.

99

LUNGE ON THE BOX

Category: Lower body strengthening, core stability.

Benefits: Strengthening of the gluteals and hamstrings, flexibility of the hip flexors, standing balance, awareness of spinal neutral.

Breathing: Inhale as your springs expand and exhale as they retract.

Variations: Hold the gondola pole for balance. The exercise can be done on reformers with legs in the same manner.

Prerequisites: Eve's lunge on the reformer.

Repetitions: 8 to 10

Springs: 1 to 2

Cues:
- Push into the front heel as you extend backward.
- Maintain neutral at the ribcage and the pelvis.
- Reach out through the crown of your head.
- Keep your ASIS square with the wall in front of you.

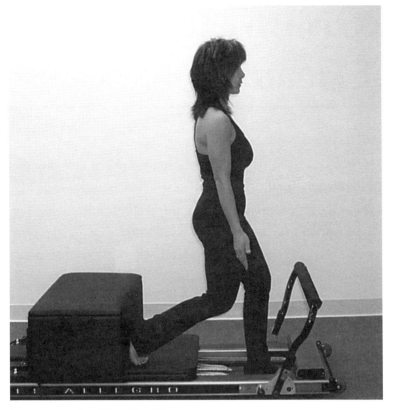

Set Up: Place the box horizontally on the carriage against the shoulder rests. Stand with your left foot on the floor inside the spring cage and your right foot against the box.

Lunge on the Box Set Up

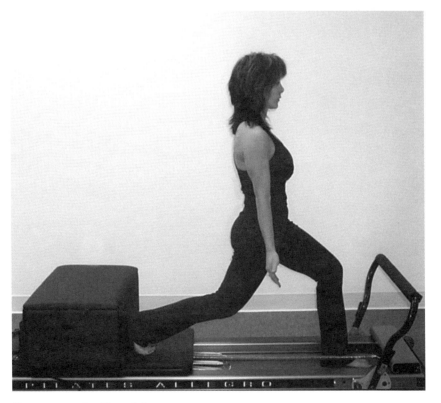

Movement: Extend the right lower extremity while keeping the left knee bent. Return the carriage home.

Lunge on the Box Movement

ROWING FRONT SERIES
Shave Back of Head

Category: Upper body strengthening, core stability.

Benefits: Strengthening of the upper body, flexibility of the lower body, lumbar and shoulder stability, breath with movement, proximal stability and distal mobility.

Breathing: Inhale as you extend your elbows and exhale as you flex them for the first 3 repetitions. Then reverse the breath to exhale on the extension for 3 repetitions.

Variations: As you become more advanced do this exercise in the long sit position (staff pose).

Prerequisites: The ability to hinge at the hips while maintaining spinal neutral. Participants should be able to perform this exercise on the mat prior to reformer work.

Repetitions: 5 to 8

Springs: 1 to 2

Cues:
- Keep your ischial tuberosities firmly on the carriage.
- Press into the carriage with your knees in the cross legged position.
- Keep the back straight and the spine stable.
- Reach long through the crown of your head.
- Keep your head in line with your spine.

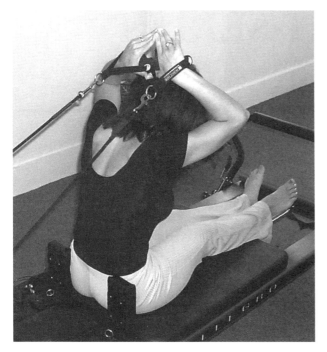

Set Up: Sit cross legged on the carriage facing the footrest with your back against the shoulder rests. Hinge forward from your hips with a straight back and hold the small loops or handles in your hands. Place your hands behind your head with your thumbs and index fingers making the shape of a diamond.

Shave Back Of Head Set Up

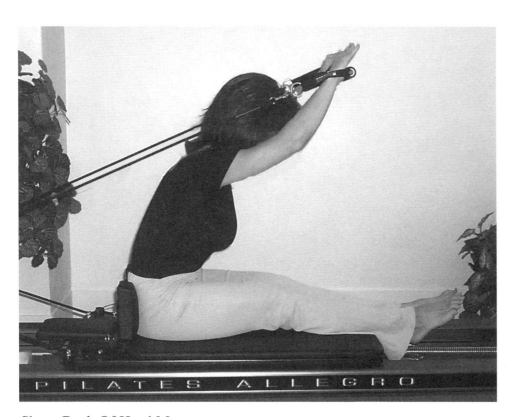

Shave Back Of Head Movement

Movement: Keep leaning forward as you extend your elbows without locking and then return to the starting position with control.

ROWING FRONT SERIES
Full Rowing Front

Category: Core stability, upper body strengthening and lower body flexibility.

Benefits: Strengthening of the upper body and powerhouse, flexibility of the upper and lower body, proximal stability and distal mobility.

Breathing: Exhale as you stretch forward, inhale as you reach your arms behind. Inhale to float the torso up and exhale as you circle your arms back to the beginning position.

Variations: For beginners try breaking the movement into pieces before completing the full exercise.

Prerequisites: Chest out down, salute, and shave back of head on the reformer.

Repetitions: 5 to 8

Springs: 1 to 2

Cues:
- Stay on the ischial tuberosities as you stretch forward.
- Do not allow the hands to extend behind the shoulders on the circle.
- Maintain the head as a natural extension of the spine.
- Maintain a "C" curve when extended forward.
- As you re-stack, follow your fingers with your eyes.

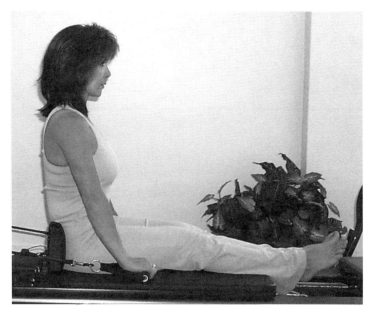

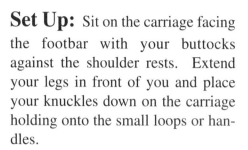

Set Up: Sit on the carriage facing the footbar with your buttocks against the shoulder rests. Extend your legs in front of you and place your knuckles down on the carriage holding onto the small loops or handles.

Rowing Front Set Up

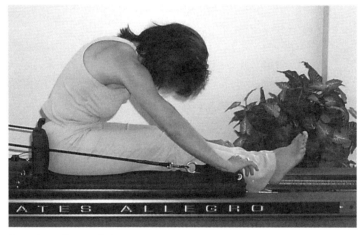

Rowing Front Movement

Movement: Begin by reaching your hands toward your feet and rounding the spine into a "C" curve. Reach out into the handles and draw your shoulder blades down as you restack the vertebrae into a hinged forward long sit position (carriage will remain still during this motion). To complete the motion, sit up from your hips while maintaining a straight spine and bring your arms around in a circle to the starting position on top of the carriage.

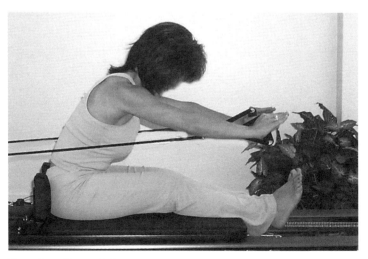

Rowing Front Movement

ROWING BACK SERIES
Full Rowing Back

Category: Core and upper body strengthening.

Benefits: Strengthening of the upper body, flexibility of the upper and lower body, proximal stability before distal mobility.

Breathing: Exhale as you roll backward, inhale as you reach your arms out. Exhale as you stretch and reach your arms forward. Inhale while you return to the beginning position.

Variations: For beginners, do not bring the arms behind. Break the movement into pieces before including all parts as a complete movement.

Prerequisites: Roll up and spine stretch on the mat. Basic rowing back on the reformer.

Repetitions: 5 to 8

Springs: 1 to 2

Cues:
- Draw your navel toward your spine as you roll backward toward the carriage.
- Stay on your ischial tuberosities as you stretch both backward and forward.
- Maintain your head as a natural extension of the spine.
- Maintain a "C" curve when extended forward.
- Keep your shoulder blades down and flat on your back when your arms are extended.

Set Up: Sit on the carriage facing the shoulder rests with your legs extended through the shoulder rests onto the head rest. Sit one hand width away from the end of the carriage. Grasp the small loops with both hands and sit tall with your spine in neutral.

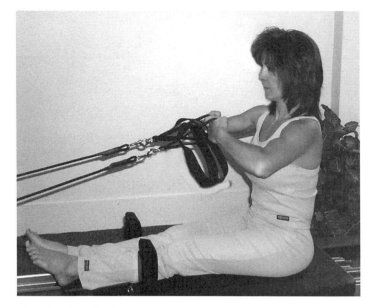

Rowing Back Set Up

Movement: Place your hands to your sternum with your knuckles together. Start rolling your spine backward toward the carriage one vertebrae at a time. When you have gone back as far as you can without losing the round back, open your arms away from your chest. Extend your arms and begin rounding the spine forward. Reach your arms behind you once you have attained a "C" curve in your spine. To complete the stretch, bring your hands forward and reach your fingers toward your feet. Return to the starting position by stacking your vertebrae one at a time.

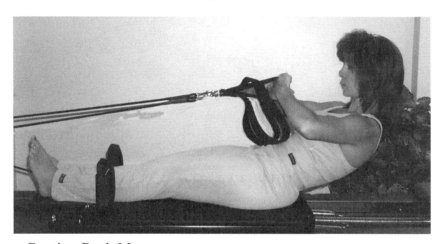

Rowing Back Movement

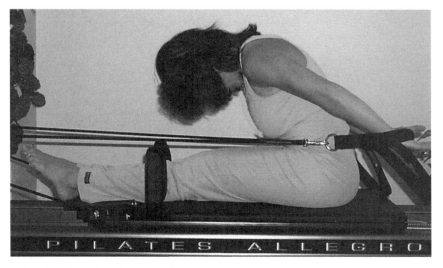

Rowing Back Movement

TWIST

Category: Core strengthening, upper body flexibility.

Benefits: Flexibility and strengthening of the upper body, strengthening of the obliques, awareness of spinal neutral in a seated position, breath with movement.

Breathing: Inhale as you move the carriage back and exhale as you return home.

Variations: To decrease difficulty, place your hands on your ribcage to feel it rotate. To increase difficulty add three pulses as you twist.

Prerequisites: Twist on the mat while in staff pose.

Repetitions: 5 to 8

Springs: 1 to 2

Cues:
- Keep the knees over the second toes and heels lifted.
- Zip the inner thighs together as you press back.
- Keep shoulders over the hips through the movement.
- Use the obliques to twist the spine to one side and then the next.
- Rotate the ribs against the pelvis.
- Stay tall through the crown of your head.
- Feel as if you "grow" through your spine during the movement.

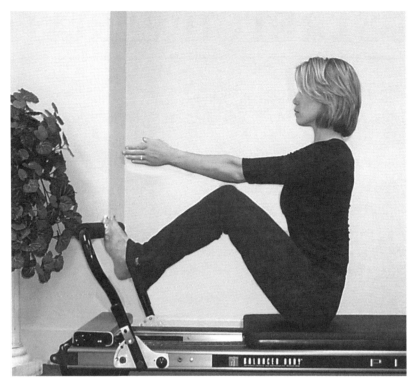
Twist Set Up

Set Up: Sit on the carriage with your feet in "Pilates V" and the balls of the feet on the foot-bar. Sit as close to the footbar as you can comfortably with a straight spine. Align the shoulders over the hips. Extend your arms in front of you with the palms together.

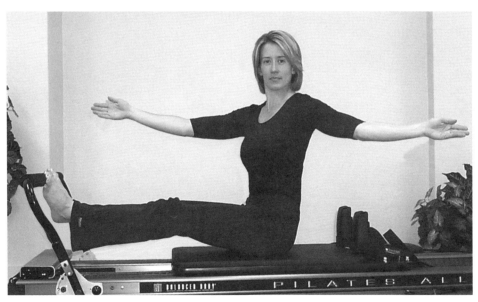
Twist Movement

Movement: Push the carriage back without locking the knees and wrap and zip your legs together. As carriage is going back arms are opening and the ribcage twists to one side. Return home, and then repeat on the other side.

KNEE STRETCH VARIATION

Category: Core stability and strengthening.

Benefits: Abdominal strengthening, flexibility of the spine, proximal stability and distal mobility, breath with movement.

Breathing: Inhale as you press backward, and exhale as you return the carriage.

Variations: For beginners, break the movement up into pieces before performing as one complete movement. For more advanced, raise the knees off of the carriage while maintaining the round back. Less springs will be more difficult.

Prerequisites: Cat on the mat. Knee stretch series on the reformer.

Repetitions: 8 to 10

Springs: 0 to 4

Cues:
- Keep your spine rounded as you perform the movements.
- Heels of your feet should be directly aligned behind your knees.
- Keep your head in line with your spine, and eyes looking downward.
- Teach as a four part movement.

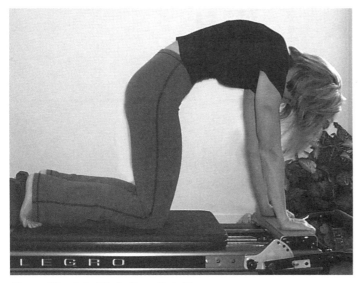

Knee Stretch Variation Set Up

Set Up: Place the footbar in the lowest position. Kneel on the carriage with your feet against the shoulder rests and your hands on the sandy surface. Draw your navel to your spine and round your back.

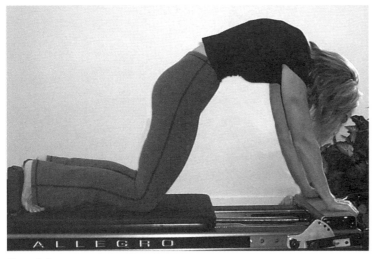

Leg Movement

Movement: Begin by pushing your knees back past your hips. Hold your knees in this position, and push the carriage back with your arms. To return bring the knees back, then pull back with the arms.

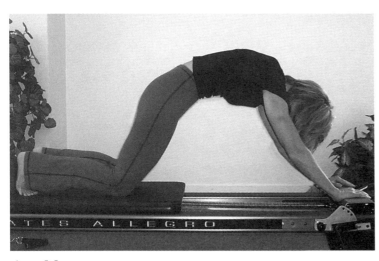

Arm Movement

KNEELING ARM SERIES
Side

Category: Core stability, upper body strengthening.

Benefits: Proximal stability and distal mobility, strengthening of the powerhouse, and upper body strengthening.

Breathing: Inhale as you reach your hand to the ceiling, exhale as you return the carriage.

Variations: For beginners, break the movement up into pieces before doing the entire movement as one complete exercise. As you become more advanced, move away from the shoulder rests.

Prerequisites: Side plank series on the mat. Kneeling arms series and rowing front and back on the reformer.

Repetitions: 5 to 8

Springs: 1 to 2

Cues:
- Keep the tailbone between your legs with the pelvis and ribcage in neutral during the entire movement.
- Do not allow your shoulder to elevate as you extend your arm to the ceiling.
- Reach out of the crown of your head to lengthen your neck as you perform the exercise.
- Align your heels directly behind your knees.

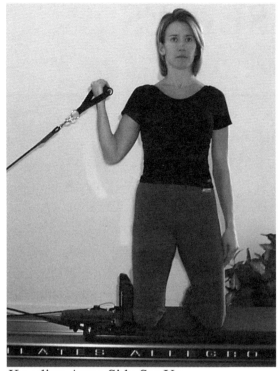

Set Up: Kneel on the carriage sideways with the side of your lower leg against the shoulder rests. Knees hip width apart. Grasp one handle with the palm up and draw your elbow into your side.

Kneeling Arms Side Set Up

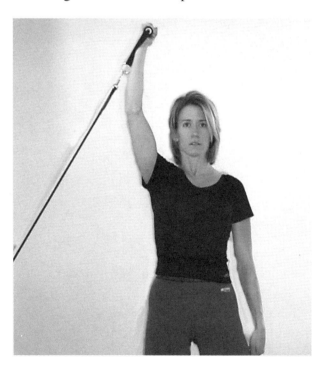

Kneeling Arms Side Beginning Movement

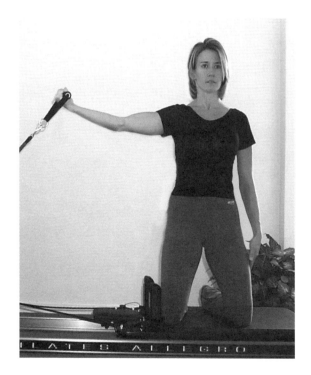

Kneeling Arms Side End Movement

Movement: Reach your hand to the ceiling, keeping your shoulders down and spine in neutral. Lower your arm to shoulder height with the elbow extended, and then flex the elbow to draw your arm back to your side.

KNEELING ARM SERIES
Circles

Category: Core stability, upper body strengthening and flexibility.

Benefits: Strengthening and stability of the Powerhouse, balance, and awareness of neutral in kneeling.

Breathing: Inhale as you start to circle, and exhale as you bring your arms back to the beginning.

Variations: For beginners, break the movement up into pieces or stick to smaller circles. For shoulder instability, shorten the lever length by drawing the elbow into the ribcage. More advanced participants can kneel with their feet away from the shoulder rests. Try reversing the direction.

Prerequisites: Chest out down and rowing arms front on the reformer.

Repetitions: 5 to 8

Springs: 1 to 2

Cues:

- Keep the tailbone between your legs with pelvis and ribcage in neutral during the entire movement.
- Do not allow your shoulders to elevate as your arms circle.
- Reach out of the crown of your head to lengthen your neck as you perform the exercise.
- Reach through your arms and protract your shoulder blades as you circle.

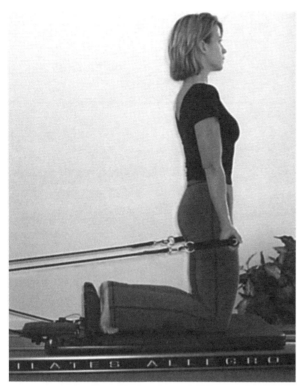

Kneeling Arm Circles Set Up

Set Up: Kneel on the carriage facing the footbar with the feet against the shoulder rests. The pelvis and ribcage are in neutral with your tailbone between your legs. Place your hands in the small loops or handles at your sides.

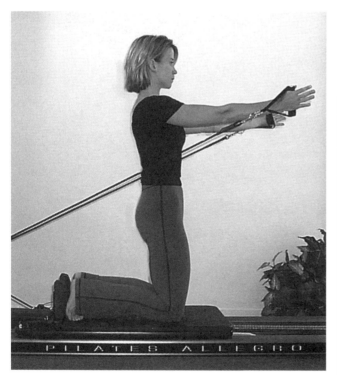

Kneeling Arm Circles Movement

Movement: While maintaining alignment bring the arms around in a circle without allowing your hands to pass behind your shoulders.

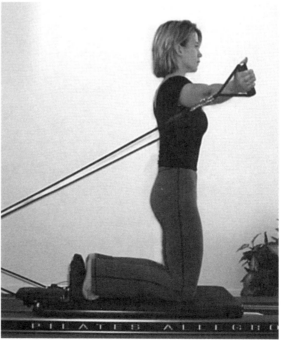

Kneeling Arm Circles Movement

KNEELING ARM SERIES
Back

Category: Core stability, upper body strengthening and flexibility.

Benefits: Strengthening and stability in the Powerhouse, balance, awareness of neutral spine in kneeling, and upper extremity strengthening.

Breathing: Inhale as you pull your straps, and exhale as you return your arms to the starting position.

Variations: Try this same exercise performing an upright row motion. For more variety and upper body strengthening, bring your elbows up to shoulder height with your palms facing you. Once in this position, stabilize your core and perform a bicep curl. Try to keep your elbows in line with your shoulders. As you become more advanced, move your feet away from the shoulder rests and kneel in the center of the carriage with your toes curled over the front edge of the carriage.

Prerequisites: Chest expansion on the reformer.

Repetitions: 5 to 8

Springs: 1 to 2

Cues:
- Keep the tailbone between your legs, and pelvis and ribcage in neutral during the entire movement.
- Do not allow your back to arch as you pull the straps.
- Reach out of the crown of your head to lengthen your neck as you perform the exercise.

Set Up: Kneel on the carriage facing the back of the reformer with the knees against the shoulder rests. Place the pelvis and ribcage in neutral with your tailbone between your legs. Place your hands in the handles, elbows extended, and palms toward the footbar.

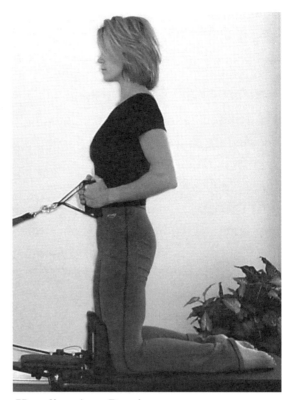

Kneeling Arm Rowing

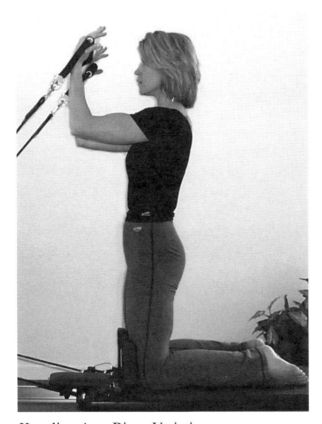

Kneeling Arm Bicep Variation

Movement: Flex the elbows with the hands supinating drawing the arms backward in a rowing motion. Keep the arms along your sides and return to the starting position.

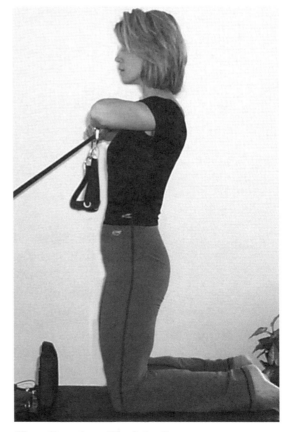

Kneeling Arm Upright Row

THIGH STRETCH

Category: Core stability and strengthening, spine and lower body flexibility.

Benefits: Powerhouse strengthening, flexibility of the spine and lower extremities, breath with movement.

Breathing: Exhale as you hinge backward, pause and inhale, then exhale to return to the starting position.

Variations: To make this exercise more difficult kneel in the middle of the carriage with toes curled around the front edge of the carriage. The footbar may need to be lowered for some in this position. To assist beginners use heavier springs.

Prerequisites: Leg pull front on mat. Kneeling arms back and short box straight back on the reformer.

Repetitions: 3 to 5

Springs: 1 to 2

Cues:

- Keep your tailbone between your legs while in kneeling position.
- Do not lead with your head, keep it as a natural extension of the spine.
- Do not allow spine to move from neutral as you arch backward; stay in a range of motion where you can maintain spinal neutral.
- Heels of your feet should be directly aligned behind your knees.
- Navel to spine to support as you hinge forward and back.

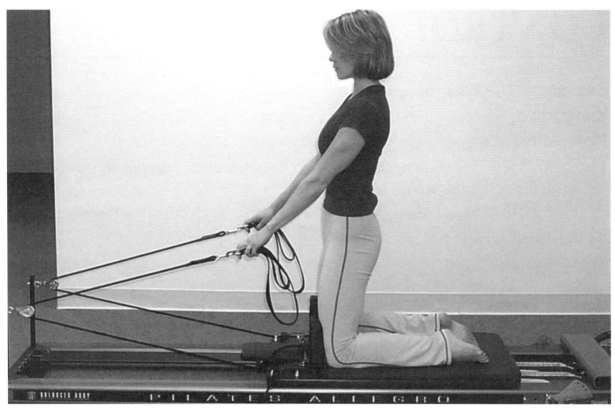

Thigh Stretch Set Up

Set Up: Kneel on the carriage with your knees against the shoulder rests, hold onto the loops with your fingers through the d-ring.

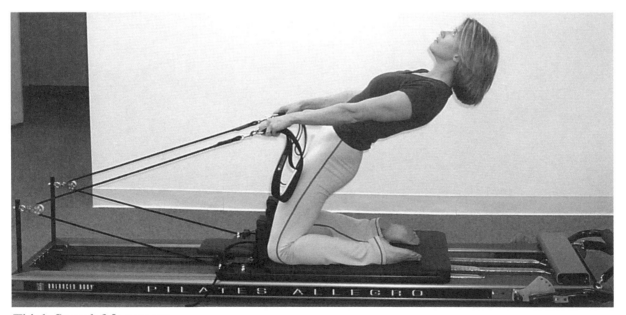

Thigh Stretch Movement

Movement: Start in kneeling position, then begin by hinging your torso toward the footbar while using the ropes for support. Lower your upper body back as far as you comfortably can while still keeping the pelvis and ribcage in neutral. Bring your torso back up to the straight back kneeling position.

CONTROL FRONT

Category: Upper body strengthening and core stability.

Benefits: Strengthening of the powerhouse and upper body.

Breathing: Inhale as you push the carriage back and exhale as you return.

Variations: To increase the difficulty, place your feet closer together on the footbar in "Pilates V" or lift one foot behind, in arabesque.

Prerequisites: Leg pull front on the mat. Long stretch and upstretch on the reformer.

Repetitions: 3 to 5

Springs: 1 to 2

Cues:
- Keep your hands below shoulder height to avoid strain to the shoulders.
- Hold spinal neutral as you perform the exercise.
- Avoid hyperextension of the elbows and knees.
- Reach out through the crown of your head.
- Maintain a wide back without winging of the shoulder blades.

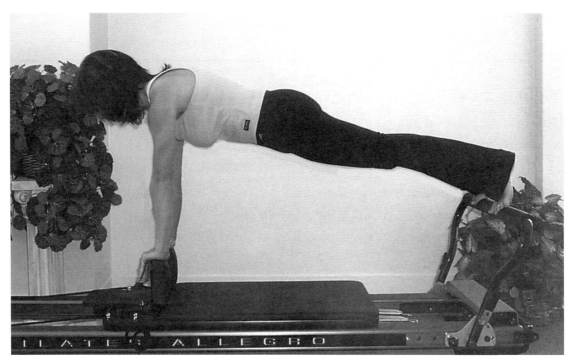

Control Front Set Up

Set Up: Get into a plank position with your hands on the shoulder rests and your feet hip width apart on the footbar.

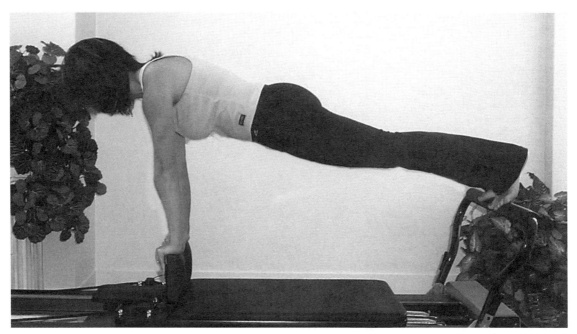

Control Front Movement

Movement: Slide the carriage in and out with your shoulders as you maintain the plank position. Emphasize the motion of bringing your hands underneath you.

GONDOLA I

Category: Core stability, lower body strengthening and flexibility.

Benefits: Powerhouse stability, strengthening of the lower extremities, especially the hip abductors and adductors, and flexibility of the hip.

Breathing: Inhale as you push the carriage back and exhale as you return.

Variations: For beginners, narrow the stance on the carriage. As participants progress, allow them to do the movement without using the gondola pole.

Prerequisites: Plie and leg circles on the mat. Side split and leg circles on the reformer.

Repetitions: 3 to 5

Springs: 1 to 2

Cues:
- Maintain neutral pelvis while performing the movement.
- Engage your pelvic floor to keep your tailbone between your legs.
- Keep spine in neutral with ribcage directly above and in line with your pelvis.
- Reach out of the crown of your head.
- Do not hyperextend the knees.

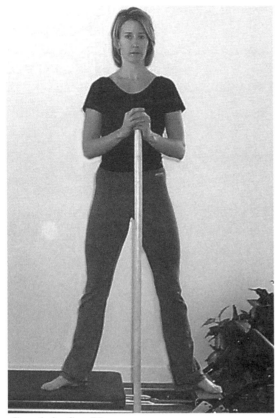

Gondola Set Up

Set Up: Stand sideways on the reformer with one foot on the sandy surface and the other against the shoulder rest. Align your feet with one another and rotate your hips outward. Position your pelvis in neutral with the ASIS and pubic symphysis in line with the wall in front of you. Hold onto a gondola pole to help yourself balance during the movement.

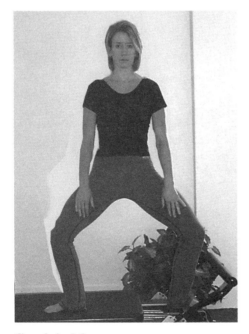

Gondola Movement

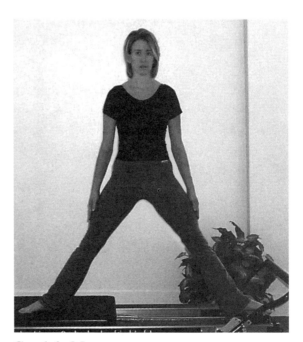

Gondola Movement

Movement: While keeping the carriage parked, perform a plie with the knees going over the second toes and the spine in neutral. From the plie position, extend both knees pushing the carriage out and then return to park with knees extended.

GONDOLA II

Category: Powerhouse stability, lower body strengthening.

Benefits: Powerhouse stability, strengthening of the lower extremities, especially the hip abductors and adductors, flexibility of the hip.

Breathing: Inhale as you push the carriage back and exhale as you return.

Variations: As participants progress, they can perform the exercise without holding onto the gondola pole, and stand with feet wider apart on the carriage.

Prerequisites: Plie on the mat. Side split and gondola I on the reformer.

Repetitions: 3 to 5

Springs: 1 to 2

Cues:
- Engage the pelvic floor to keep your tailbone between your legs.
- Keep spine in neutral with ribcage directly in line with your pelvis.

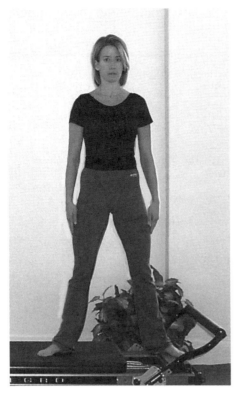

Set Up: Stand with feet hip width apart, one foot on the sandy surface and the other on the carriage. Align your feet with one another, and externally rotate your hips. Place pelvis in neutral with the ASIS and pubic symphysis in line with the wall in front of you. Hold onto a gondola pole to help yourself balance during the movement.

Gondola II Set Up

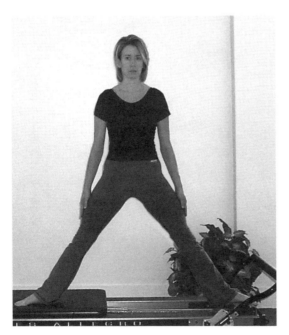

Gondola II Movement

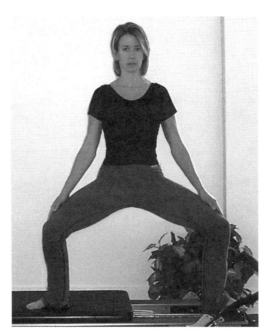

Gondola II Movement

Movement: Push your carriage out by abducting both legs and keep the knees extended. Once you are in the split position, draw the carriage back to park by bending your knees into a plie. Straighten your knees once the carriage is parked.

JUMPBOARD

Category: Lower extremity strengthening.

Benefits: Increased lower extremity strength and power, plyometric training, increased powerhouse stability, anaerobic training.

Breathing: Inhale as you jump, exhale as you return.

Variations: Change the foot position to plie' narrow, plie' wide, hip width, high or low on the pad, etc. Change the jump to accommodate crossing of the lower extremities, straddle or split. Hold the bent knee position with the feet low on the pad to stretch the anterior tibialis. When you have mastered the supine position try the jump in side lying.

Prerequisites: Footwork in neutral spine.

Repetitions: 3 to 5

Springs: 3 to 4

Cues:
- Maintain a neutral spine throughout.
- Land quietly.
- For a plyometric effect rebound immediately on landing.

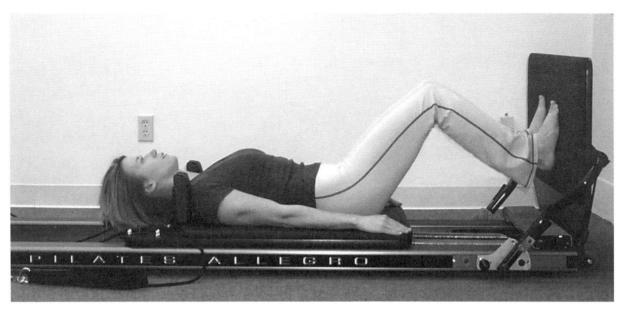

Jumpboard Set Up

Set Up: Place the jumpboard on the reformer. Lie supine with your feet hip width apart as low on the jump board as you can with your heels down. Stay in neutral spine.

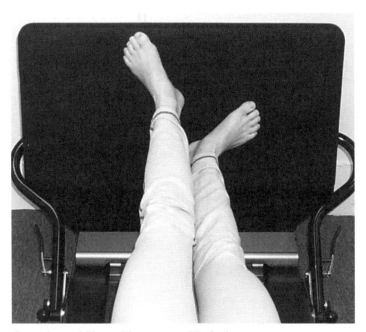

Jumpboard Foot Placement Variation

Movement: Jump by pushing off the jump board and maintain a neutral spine as you return and jump again. Try the listed variations or create jumps related to the client's sport.

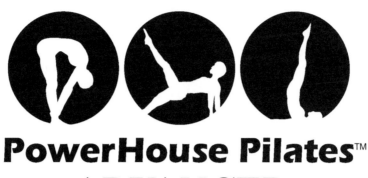

PowerHouse Pilates™
ADVANCED
REFORMER EXERCISES

This section is designed to introduce you to more complex Pilates reformer exercises. There are many more advanced exercises, but we selected only a few for you to experience. After your body feels comfortable with the first two sections of this book, experiment gradually with the advanced exercises in your own workout routine.

These exercises are not recommended for group Pilates Reformer classes. They should only be taught to experienced clientele in a personal training session. Be careful to keep the number of repetitions low and the movement precise to avoid injury.

"Be certain that you have your entire body under complete mental control."
Joseph Pilates

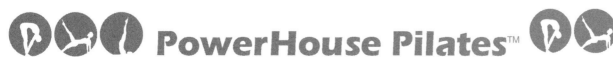
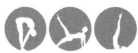

CORKSCREW

Category: Core strengthening.

Benefits: Abdominal strengthening, flexibility of the spine, breath with movement.

Breathing: Inhale as you extend your legs to the ceiling, and exhale as you roll back onto the carriage. Inhale in the rolled position and exhale as you return to the starting position.

Variations: Bend your knees toward your chest, as in short spine, and roll down with your knees on your chest.

Prerequisites: Rollover and rolling like a ball on mat. Short spine and long spine on the reformer.

Repetitions: 8 to 10

Springs: Not applicable as carriage does not move.

Cues:
- Squeeze the lower extremities together to draw in the deep abdominal muscles.
- Do not roll onto your neck.
- Widen the back and soften the neck.
- Keep distance between your thighs and torso.

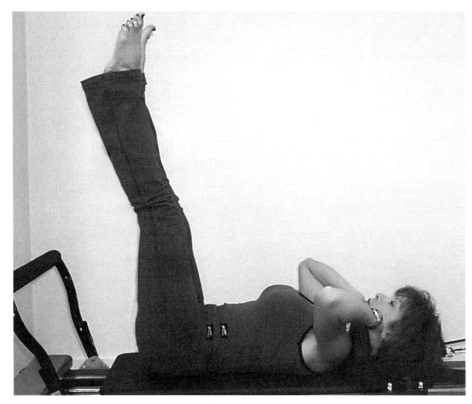

Corkscrew Set Up

Set Up: Lie supine on the carriage with the head rest down, the pelvis and ribcage in neutral and the lower extremities extended toward the ceiling. Hold the shoulder posts with your hands.

Movement: The carriage will remain in the parked position for this exercise. Draw your navel to your spine and peel your vertebrae from the carriage starting at the sacrum and extending to the to the shoulder blades. As you roll, go off to one side of the spinal column. Allow your feet to extend over your face, but do not roll onto your neck. Roll back down to the carriage with control on the same side of the spine. Then repeat on the other side.

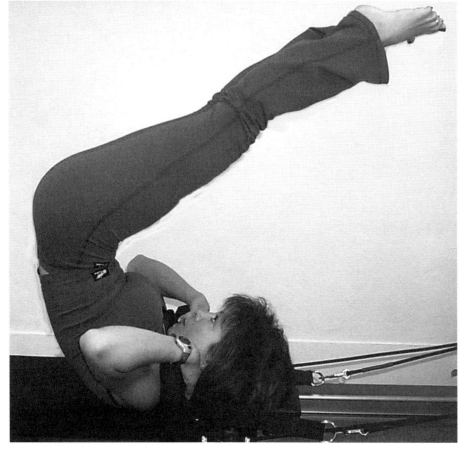

Corkscrew Movement

131

LONG BACK STRETCH

Category: Upper body strengthening.

Benefits: Strengthening of the upper body, core stability, pectoralis minor, stretch, breath with movement, proximal stability and distal mobility.

Breathing: Inhale as you move the carriage back and exhale as you return home.

Variations: Do the exercise three times in this order and then reverse the motion for three repetitions. For beginners, break the motion into pieces. For shorter individuals, use a block or bring the footbar closer.

Prerequisites: Reverse plank and table top on the mat.

Repetitions: 8 to 10

Springs: 1 to 2

Cues:
- Avoid hyperextension of the knees and elbows.
- Widen the back and soften the neck.
- Keep the shoulder blades down the back.
- Try to maintain a neutral wrist.
- Keep neutral spinal alignment throughout the movement.

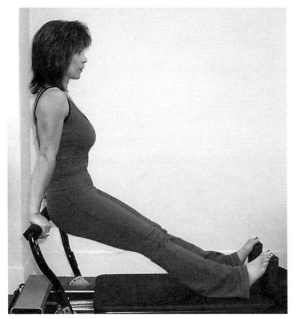

Long Back Stretch Set Up

Set Up: Place your hands on the footbar and your feet against the shoulder rests in a long sit position. Be sure to pronate your hands with your palms facing backward, your back straight, your hips flexed, and your buttocks close to the footbar.

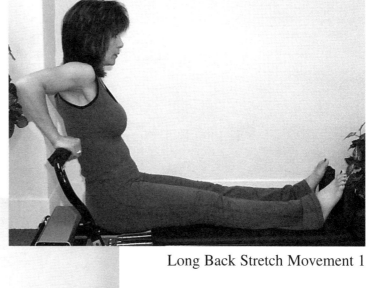

Long Back Stretch Movement 1

Movement: With the carriage parked, bend your elbows dropping your buttocks toward the springs and then push the carriage back by extending the elbows. Hold the carriage in this position as you raise your buttocks and extend your spine with the elbows extended. Return to the starting position by performing shoulder flexion back to midline.

Long Back Stretch Movement 2

RUSSIAN SPLIT

Category: Lower body strengthening, core stability.

Benefits: Flexibility and strengthening of the lower body, balance and powerhouse stability.

Breathing: Inhale as you move the carriage back and exhale as you return home.

Variations: Try the lunge pressing out with the front leg bent and returning with the front leg straight. To strengthen the Vastus Medialis, hold the lunge and extend and flex the front knee with control. As balance and strength improves put all the motions together into a four part series. For those who cannot balance on the footbar, have them place their back foot onto the sandy surface in external rotation or use the gondola pole.

Prerequisites: Eve's lunge and gondola series on the reformer.

Repetitions: 8 to 10

Springs: 1 to 2

Cues:
- Keep your ASIS square with the wall in front of you.
- Avoid hyperextension of the knees.
- Reach tall through the crown of your head.
- Keep your tailbone between your legs during the movement.
- Maintain ribcage and pelvis alignment.

Set Up: Stand on the carriage with one foot on the footbar and the other toward the head rest. Align your patella with your second toe and flex your front knee. Press out until your knee is aligned directly over your ankle. Keep the tail bone pointing down, the pelvis and spine in neutral, and your pelvis aligned with the wall in front of you. Hold onto a gondola pole if needed for balance.

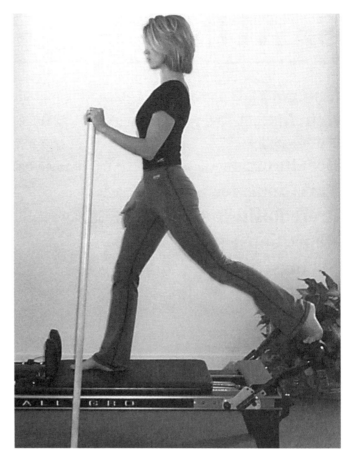

Russian Split Set Up

Movement: Push the carriage back, moving into a lunge position. Return the carriage with control to the starting position.

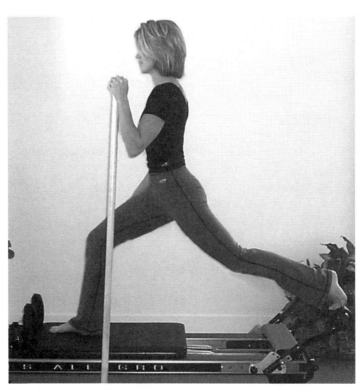

Russian Split Movement

SKATING

Category: Lower body strengthening, core stability.

Benefits: Flexibility and strengthening of the lower body, balance and coordination, powerhouse stability.

Breathing: Inhale as you move the carriage back and exhale as you return home.

Variations: For beginners, place the feet more narrow on the carriage.

Prerequisites: Side split and gondola series on the reformer.

Repetitions: 8 to 10

Springs: 1 to 2

Cues:

- Avoid hyperextension of the knees.
- Reach tall through the crown of your head.
- Feel a wrapping sensation in the buttocks as you draw your legs together.
- Widen the back and soften the neck.
- Keep the turn out coming from the hip joints.

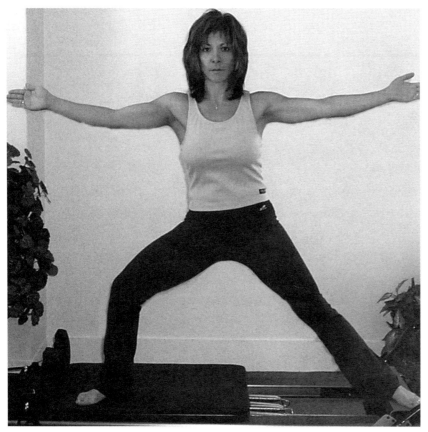

Skate Set Up

Set Up: Stand on the carriage with one foot on the sandy surface of the footplate and the other against the shoulder rest. Align your second toes with your patellae and place your hips in slight external rotation. Keep the tail bone pointing down and the pelvis and spine in neutral. Hold your arms in front of you or hold the gondola to assist with balance.

Movement: Push the carriage back, using the leg on the carriage and bending the knee as if you were lunging into the carriage. Then return the carriage with control as you internally rotate the hip of the leg on the carriage and bend the knee of the leg on the foot plate. While your legs are pressing back and forth, reach your arms out for balance. Keep this back and forth movement without bringing the carriage to park, just as if you were skating or rollerblading.

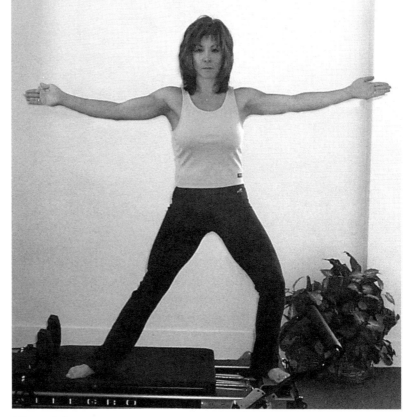

Skate Movement

137

SNAKE

Category: Core strengthening, upper body strengthening and flexibility.

Benefits: Increase powerhouse and upper body strength, increase shoulder stability, and increase torso flexibility.

Breathing: Inhale as you move the carriage back and exhale as you return home.

Variations: For more advanced participants, place the hands shoulder width apart on the carriage with one hand on the shoulder rest and one on the side of the carriage. For beginners, perform this exercise on the mat until they are strong enough for the reformer.

Prerequisites: Control front, long stretch, and mermaid on the reformer. Snake, twist, and side plank on the mat.

Repetitions: 8 to 10

Springs: 1 to 2

Cues:
- Keep the ASIS's facing the carriage when the carriage is pushed out.
- Elongate the spine as you extend.
- Widen the back and soften the neck.
- Draw the navel to the spine in the extended position.
- Make sure not to compress your low back.
- Keep your feet twisted when the carriage is in the pushed out position.

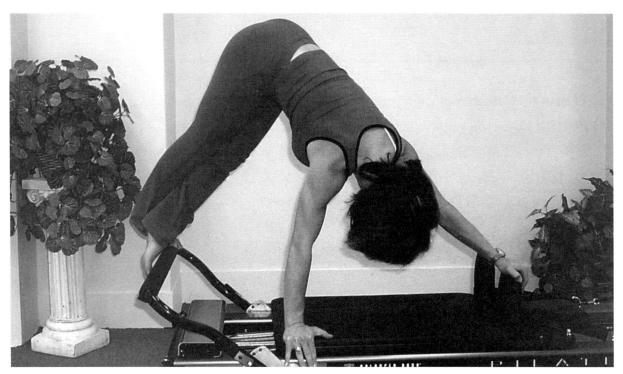

Snake Set Up

Set Up: While facing the right side of the carriage, place your left foot on the outer edge of the footbar with your right foot crossed over it. Place your right hand on the opposite shoulder rest and your left hand on the front edge of the carriage. Pike your buttocks upward and draw your chest toward your thighs. Keep your knees and elbows softly extended.

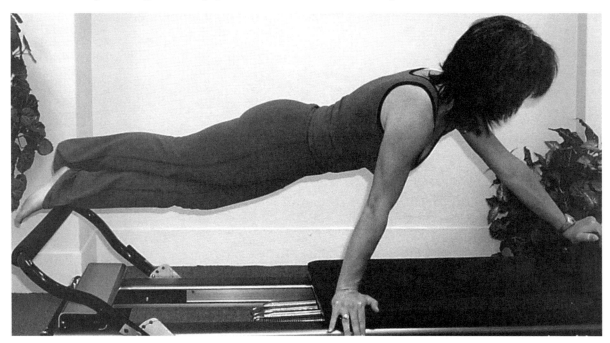

Snake Movement

Movement: Push the carriage back, as you extend your hips and and spine to look toward the rope pulleys and align the pelvis with the carriage. After you have fully extended, return to the starting position with control, resisting the pull of the springs.

STAR

Category: Core strengthening and stability, upper body strengthening.

Benefits: Strengthening of the powerhouse, unilateral strengthening of the upper body.

Breathing: Inhale as you push out, and exhale as you draw back toward the footbar.

Variations: For beginners to attain the balance and stability, allow them to hold the position only. It is often helpful to add heavier springs. As you progress, separate the legs hip width and reach the top arm to the ceiling. Keep this position as you push the carriage out and return.

Prerequisites: Side plank and star on the mat. Mermaid on the reformer.

Repetitions: 3 to 5

Springs: 1 to 2

Cues:
- Keep spinal and pelvic neutral while you push in and out with the supporting arm.
- Do not allow the torso to twist or bend.
- Keep your neck as a natural extension of your spine and reach out of the crown of your head.
- Do not allow the weight bearing scapula to elevate.

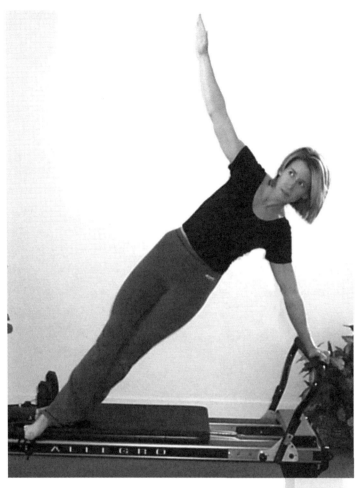

Star Set Up

Set Up: Place one hand on the footbar with your knuckles away from the carriage, and your fingers and thumb together. Place the bottom foot against the shoulder rest in a flexed position and stack the other foot on top. Align the shoulders and hips with the wall in front of you and place your top hand on your hip.

Movement: Push the carriage away from the footbar while maintaining alignment. Then return the carriage.

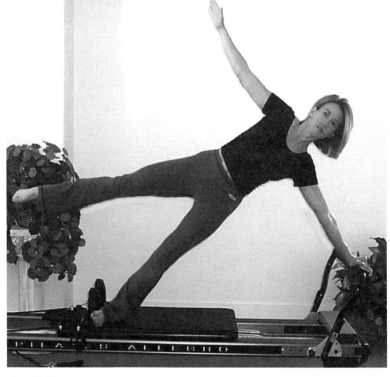

Star Movement

141

TENDON STRETCH

Category: Upper body strengthening, spine flexibility, core strengthening and stability.

Benefits: Abdominal and upper body strengthening, flexibility of the spine, breath with movement.

Breathing: Inhale as you push your feet forward, and exhale as you move back into the pike position.

Variations: For someone with very tight hamstrings, maintain spinal alignment and bend slightly at the knees. Beginners can work to attain the set up position or push only through the movement portion before trying the entire exercise.

Prerequisites: Elephant, arabesque, and long back stretch on the reformer.

Repetitions: 3 to 5

Springs: 1 to 2

Cues:

- Keep your spine round throughout the movement.
- Do not allow your shoulder blades to elevate toward your ears when in the weight bearing position of the exercise.
- Keep your head as a natural extension of your spine; avoid raising your chin when pushing forward.
- Keep your ischial tuberosities to the ceiling in the beginning phase of the exercise.

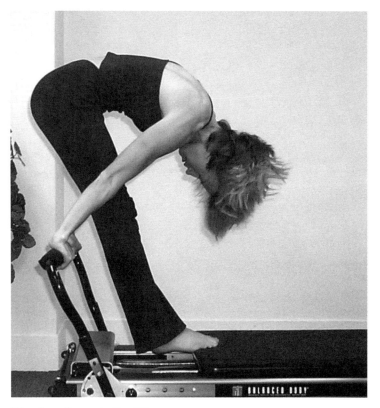

Tendon Stretch Set Up

Set Up: Sit on the footbar facing the carriage. Place your hands shoulder width apart on the footbar with your knuckles facing the carriage. Place the balls of your feet on the edge of the carriage and keep your legs together. Lift your buttocks and round your spine with your ischial tuberosities toward the ceiling in a pike position.

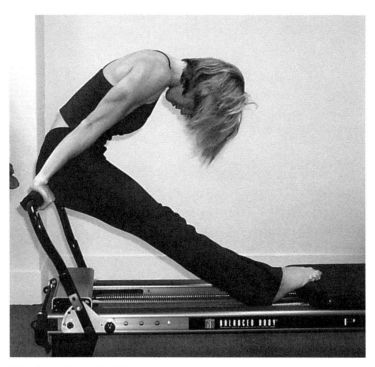

Tendon Stretch Movement

Movement: From the pike position, push the carriage out with your feet while bringing your torso between your arms. Push out only until your torso is in line with your arms, then engage your abdominals to return to the pike position.

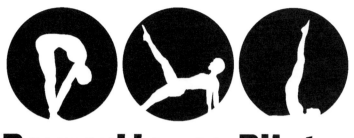

PowerHouse Pilates™

BEGINNING YOUR OWN
PILATES PROGRAM

This section contains everything from sample classes and teaching tips to health history forms and promotional flyers to assist you in planning your program. It is important to educate your entire staff on the components and benefits of Pilates exercise so that they may effectively communicate with your clientele. The most successful programs involve an integrated sales team with an appointed Pilates specialist who is available for more in-depth explanation.

"Remember, too, that "Rome was not built in a day," and that patience and persistence are vital qualities in the ultimate successful accomplishment of any worthwhile endeavor."

Joseph Pilates

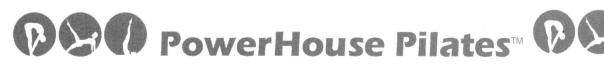
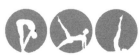

Group Reformer
Class Format (1 Hour)

We recommend one instructor to every five participants, and that the instructor does not perform the exercises with the group.

I.   **The warm-up** – will include exercises such as the hundred and footwork variations as well as breathing and pelvic neutral.   10 minutes

II. **The work-out** – will include exercises emphasizing core, lower extremity, and upper extremity strengthening and flexibility. The exercises are known for their ability to lengthen and strengthen at the same time. Examples include: stomach massage series, knee stretch, elephant, long stretch, mermaid, tree hug, rowing front and back, etc.   40 minutes

III. **The cool down** – will incorporate running mermaid and variations of footwork.

Group Reformer Teaching Tips

1. Cueing is essential. Try to use body language, imagery, and touch. Different personalities respond to different cues. Some are visual, some are verbal. Try to give many types of cues to meet the needs of the group. Experiment and see what gets the desired result.
2. Don't hesitate to use a participant as an example of proper form or successful execution of an exercise. This not only boosts confidence, but gives others a visual presentation to follow.
3. Encourage the class to look at themselves and use the mirrors. Now they have two teachers, you and themselves.
4. Always use a microphone. When you walk around and assist, you will often turn away from the class and your voice will fade.
5. Use only music without a pronounced beat. Exercises are never done to the music.
6. Try to keep a cadence with your voice. "Inhale as you press back and exhale as you return.......Inhale and zip your thighs together, keep your knees over your second toe as you return." Give as much of the instruction as possible to the general group. Avoid closing in on just one person unless he or she are in danger. Instead direct your cues to the entire group, while touching, making eye contact with, or creating a visual for the person in need of assistance.
7. If working in a team, never take a member of the class in a direction different than the lead instructor. Give enough cues to guide but avoid distracting the participant from the flow of the class.
8. Remember that in a group progress will be slower. Keep this in mind when assessing your students. What you would expect one-on-one in a single session may take 3 sessions in a group.
9. Group reformer classes will not always be appropriate for everyone. Don't hesitate to suggest to some participants that they may be more successful or safer in a private session. For some a few private sessions will be all they need to gain the ability to follow in a group successfully.

Beginner Reformer Workouts

Workout #1
Breathing and neutral spine position
Footwork I balls on feet straight – break it up 8 leg press, 8 calf raise
Footwork I pilates "V" – combined movement 8
Articulating bridge x 4 with carriage home
Pelvic lift x 8 lifted
Hundreds - knees bent 10 sets of 10
Coordination x 5 – just base move
Arm circles - 5 each direction
Leg circles – 5 each direction
Stomach massage round and flat and hamstring stretch (8 of each)
Rowing front tree hug x 6 and shave head x 6
Chest Expansion x 8
Down stretch x 8 (4 with 2 springs and 4 with 1 spring)
Knee stretch series round or knees off, and flat
Long stretch (4 with 2 springs and 4 with 1 spring)
Eve's Lunge – 5 on each side
Footwork II bird on a perch x 8
Running – 8 pushing from ankle and 8 pushing from knee

Workout #2
Footwork I parallel, press out and in 8-10 reps
Footwork I as above heels under and calf raise 8-10 reps
Footwork I as above complete 8-10 reps
Footwork I in Pilates V complete 8-10 reps
Hundred with legs in table top position
Arm Circles 3-5 repetitions each direction
Leg Circles 3-5 repetitions each direction
Frog 8-10 reps
Short Spine 3-5 reps
Chest Out Down 8-10 reps
Salute 4-6 reps
Long Stretch 3-5 reps
Elephant 8-10 reps
Eve's Lunge 3-5 reps each side
Rolling Back 6-8 reps then add Bicep Curl 6-8 reps
Knee Stretch Round 6-8 reps
Knee Stretch Flat 6-8 reps
Mermaid 3 reps on each side

Intermediate Reformer Workouts

Workout #1: This class integrates beginning and intermediate exercises.

Footwork I (Single Leg)
Pelvic Lift
Leg Circles
Single Leg Frog
Stomach Massage--Round Back
Stomach Massage--Straight Back with Arms off carriage
Full Rowing Front
Elephant
Long Stretch
Upstretch
Side Split (Using the gondola)
Kneeling Arms Back
Running

Workout #2: This class is only intermediate and advanced exercises.

Single Leg Footwork I
Single Leg Frog
Short Spine
Short Box Series--Round Back
Short Box Series--Tilt/Twist
Long Box Series--Pulling Straps
Long Box Series--Backstroke
Knee Stretch Variation
Tendon Stretch
Long Back Stretch
Star
Mermaid

Intermediate Reformer Workouts

Workout #3: This class emphasizes upper body strengthening exercises.

Footwork II
Pelvic Lift
Arm Circles
Short Box Series--Horseback
Down Stretch
Knee Stretch Series--Round Back
Salute
Shave Back of the Head
Full Rowing Front
Chest Expansion
Kneeling Arms Side
Snake
Elephant

Workout #4: This class emphasizes lower body strengthening exercises.

Running
Leg Circles
Single Leg Frog
Long Spine
Knee Stretch Series--Straight Back
Knee Stretch Series--Round Back with knees off
Arabesque
Tendon Stretch
Side Split
Gondola
Russian Split
Semicircle

PILATES MEDICAL HISTORY

Medical History
The PowerHouse Institute

Today's Date:

Name:

Address:

Phone

Date of Birth: **Sex:**

Occupation

Please circle any of the following that apply:

High Blood Pressure	Heart Problems		
Diabetes	Joint Problems		
Liver Disease	Fractures	Cancer	Asthma
Night Pain	Seizures	Pregnancy	Smoker
Shortness of Breath	Recent Surgery	Chronic Illness	Scoliosis
Osteoporosis	Back Problems		

Please Circle the types of movement you have experienced:

Dance	Yoga	Martial Arts	Running	Swimming
Aerobic Dance	Team Sports	Other:		

Current Medications	**Current Therapy or Medical Care**
1.	1.
2.	2.
3.	3.

Anything else you would like to tell us:

Notes:

Registration & Waiver

Name_____

Street Address_____

City_____**State**_____**Zip**_____

Home Phone_____   **Work Phone**_____

How did you hear about our program?

_____

What types of movement have you experienced? _____Yoga _____Dance _____Ballet

_____Fitness _____Other

ACKNOWLEDGMENT OF RISK AND WAIVER OF LIABILITY

I understand that I, _____ [Print Name], will be participating in a fitness program through the [gym or studio name] that will require physical exertion. Although the most common injuries or symptoms associated with exercise involve sprains, strains, dizziness, fainting and/or discomfort in breathing, I recognize that there is a risk of serious injury (and in extreme cases, death) associated with any fitness program. Consequently, I was advised by a member of the fitness staff at the [gym or studio name] to obtain the approval of my doctor before beginning a fitness program through the [gym or studio name], and have had the opportunity to do so. Before beginning this program, I also was asked by a member of the fitness staff at the [gym or studio name] whether I have any physical or mental limitations, or whether I am taking any medications or receiving any medical treatment that might make it unsafe for me to participate in this fitness program. There is no such limitation, medication or medical treatment other than those that I have written on the attached sheet.

I understand that, by signing this statement, I am agreeing not to hold the [gym or studio name] or any of its employees, owners, agents or insurers responsible for any bodily injury or property damage that I may suffer as a result of my participation in a fitness program through the [gym or studio name], whether at the [gym or studio name], at home or elsewhere. As such, I understand and agree that the [gym or studio name], its employees, owners, agents or insurers shall not be liable for any bodily injury or property damage that may result either directly or indirectly from my participation in a fitness program through the [gym or studio name].

_____   _____
Participant's Signature   Date

Reformer Safety and Maintenance

Before beginning a class or personal training session:

1) Make sure to inspect the straps to see if they are tight in their binding, and that they are equal in length.
2) Strap posts should be locked with the lock pins.
3) Shoulder rest should be all the way in and locked with lock pins.
4) Footbar should be adjusted to each participant's height and securely locked in place.
5) Spray tracks of all machines with silicone lubricant.

Safety Points to Remember:

1) Do not allow participants to straddle the machines. Ask them to sit on the carriage from the side first.
2) Always make sure a participant's fingers are clear of the springs when they are holding onto the carriage during a movement.
3) Change carriage springs only when the carriage is parked.
4) Do not have participants stand on the carriage without assistance or holding onto a sturdy object.
5) When assisting clients with straps, be careful not to allow the ropes to fall into their face.
6) When assisting clients into leg loops, give clear instructions and keep one foot on the footbar or in strap at all times.

Care and Maintenance:

1) Keep all tracks lubricated with a silicone lube, and free and clear of dust.
2) Wash the carriage with mild detergent between usage.
3) Keep the springs free and clear of dust, hair, etc...
4) Periodically wash the hand and foot straps in mild detergent. Allow to dry before usage.

REFORMER PRE-CLASS CHECKLIST

1)_____**Are all lock pins in place in the shoulder rests?**

2)_____**Are all lock pins in place in strap posts?**

3)_____**Have all straps been checked to be equal in length?**

4)_____**Have all strap catches been checked for tightness?**

5)_____**All machines wiped and sprayed with lubricant?**

Pilates Information Sheet

What is the name Pilates?

It is actually the name of the man who invented the exercise. His name was Joseph H. Pilates and he came to America from Germany. He had started the exercises in Germany in the 1920s while working as a nurse in a prison camp. Soon after, he began training a boxer who decided to move to America and wanted Joseph to join him as his trainer.

Joseph agreed only if they would open a studio in New York for him. Thus, the New York Pilates studio was born. While in New York Joseph invented several different machines that would then assist the exerciser with the movements that he had developed. He designed eight different machines; the two main machines became known as the Reformer and The Cadillac. Through these machines he developed hundreds of exercises.

The exercises soon caught the attention of ballet dancers, and that is where they have been taught for the past 80 years. Famous dancers, such as George Balanchine and Martha Graham have used the exercises as therapy for their injuries, and adapted the exercises to fit their needs.

In the past 5-10 years many celebrities have begun using the exercises to change and shape their bodies. Most recently it has begun to filter into the health club industry, thus creating a much larger demand for exercises that are therapeutic and relaxing.

What are the types of Pilates classes?

There are the mat classes, which are similar to Yoga. However, instead of holding a static pose, as in a Yoga class the participants experience a continuous flow of movement working both the front and back of the body. There are also the Reformer classes, which are done in small groups of five with a personal trainer.

The benefits of any type of Pilates class are increased strength and overall flexibility. Most participants report that since doing Pilates exercises that they have improved posture, flatter abdominals and increased flexibility. Joseph Pilates stated that these exercises could change a person's body in 30 days if done only 10 minutes per day. Many people come to Pilates to help heal an injury, and they end up transforming their overall appearance.

To find out where you can try a Pilates class
Call the PowerHouse Institute at 1-877-716-4879

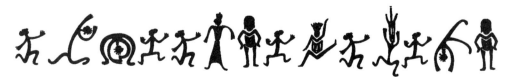

REFORM YOUR BODY

Free Introductory Classes on the

PILATES REFORMER

Thursday 7/27/00 4:30PM

Friday 7/28/00 10:30AM

Thursday 8/3/00 10:45AM

Friday 8/4/00 6:45 PM

Limited to 5 members per class.

You must register at the front desk.

Sample poster

PowerHouse Institute Class Policies and Guidelines

All class packages expire 6 months from the purchase date. We will provide you with a card that has the expiration date on it to remind you.

The mat classes are sold as 10 and 20 sessions at a discount. The single class rate is $15 for members and $25 for non-members. Class packages may not be shared by more than one participant. **We have a strict 2-hour cancellation policy for the Reformer Group Class or Personal Training sessions.** If participants fails to cancel within that time, they will be billed for that session.

All payments are made through the front desk.
All Pilates Personal Training is arranged individually with the instructor.

All non-members must pay a $10 guest fee to the fitness center when trying an introductory class.

GLOSSARY

Anterior – the front of the body.

Anterior Triangle – a line connecting the front points of the pelvis: including the bilateral ASIS and the pubic symphysis.

ASIS (Anterior Superior Iliac Spine) – the uppermost points of the iliac crests in the front of the pelvic girdle.

Atrophy - a wasting or decreasing of size of an organ or tissue.

"Boinking" – a term used to describe the ribcage when it comes out of a neutral position and the 10th rib is positioned anterior and superior to its ideal location.

"C" Curve – indicates an even gentle rounding of the spine.

Contrology – what Joseph Pilates named his method of body conditioning.

Core – the deep intrinsic muscles of the torso that support the spine.

Distal – further from the center of the body.

Down Dog – a yoga position where the hands and feet are on the floor and the hips are flexed to bring the body into a position of an upside down "V".

Extension – the act of moving into a straight condition; the angle of the joint becomes larger.

External Rotation – turning of a joint outward away from the center of the body.

Extrinsic Muscles – the outermost visible muscles of the body.

Flexion – the act of bending; the angle of the joint becomes smaller.

Girdle – a structure that resembles a circular belt or band.

Gondola Pole – a wooden rod used for balance.

Hyperextend – to extend to the extreme or abnormal extension.

Internal Rotation – turning of a joint inward toward the center of the body.

Intrinsic Muscles – the deep muscles of the body; often described as the glue.

Ischial Tuberosity – the lowest point of the ischium in the pelvic girdle on which we sit.

Mobility – state or quality of being mobile; facility of movement.

Neutral Spine – neutral pelvis plus neutral ribcage plus neutral shoulder girdle plus cervical neutral.

Pelvic Neutral – a position half way between a forward tilt of the pelvis and a backward tilt of the pelvis where the muscles about the pelvis can function with even strength and length for long periods of time.

"Pilates V" - a position of the lower extremities where the femurs are slightly externally rotated, the heels are together, the second toes are in line with the patella, and there is a wrapping sensation in the muscles of the buttocks.

Plyometric – a quick eccentric contraction of a muscle prior to the concentric contraction; an example would be repeated jumps one after the other without a pause in between.

Posterior – the back of the body.

Powerhouse – the area from your shoulder girdle to your pelvis; often referred to as the core.

Pronation – turning the foot or palm downward.

Prone – lying horizontal with the face downward.

Protract – drawing the scapula away from each other in a forward motion.

Proximal – closer to the center of the body.

"Sits" Bones - the ischial tuberosities of the ischium.

Stability – state or quality of being fixed; not moving.

Staff Pose – long sitting position where the legs are extended and the hips are at ninety degrees.

Supination – turning of the foot or palm upward.

Supine – lying on the back or with the face upward.

Widen the Back – protract and downwardly rotate the scapula.

Winging Shoulder Blades – indicates a position of the scapula where they stand away from the ribcage when the shoulder girdle is challenged.

Zip and Wrap - a cue used to create the "Pilates V" position of the lower extremities; imagine a zipper on the posterior surface of the inner thighs.